$20.00

B

# Pocket Atlas
# of Ophthalmology

D0743934

LINDA BERTRAM

Fritz Hollwich

# Pocket Atlas
# of Ophthalmology

Translated by Frederick C. Blodi

365 Colored Illustrations

1981
Georg Thieme Verlag Stuttgart · New York

Prof. Dr. Dr. h.c. F. Hollwich
Antonienstr. 1
D-8000 München 40

*Translator*
F.C. Blodi, M.D.
Prof. and Head
Dept. of Ophthalmology
University of Iowa
College of Medicine
Iowa City, Iowa, 52242
USA

**Deutsche Bibliothek Cataloguing in Publication Data**

**Hollwich, Fritz:**
Pocket atlas of ophthalmology / Fritz Hollwich. Transl. by
Frederick C. Blodi. − Stuttgart ; New York : Thieme; Chicago ; London : Year
Book Med. Publ., 1981.
   (Thieme flexibooks)
   Dt. Ausg. u.d.T.: Hollwich, Fritz: Taschenatlas der Augenheilkunde

**Important Note:**
Medicine is an ever-changing science. Research and clinical experience are continually broadening our knowledge, in particular our knowledge of proper treatment and drug therapy. Insofar as this book mentions any dosage or application, readers may rest assured that the authors, editors and publishers have made every effort to ensure that such references are strictly in accordance with the state of knowledge at the time of production of the book. Nevertheless, every user is requested to carefully examine the manufacturers' leaflets accompanying each drug to check on his own responsibility whether the dosage schedules recommended therein or the contraindications stated by the manufacturers differ from the statements made in the present book. Such examination is particularly important with drugs which are either rarely used or have been newly released on the market.

1st German edition 1980
This book is an authorized translation from the 1st revised German edition published and copyrighted 1980 by Georg Thieme Verlag, Stuttgart, Germany. Title of the German edition: Taschenatlas der Augenheilkunde.
Some of the product names, patents and registered designs referred to in this book are in fact registered trademarks or proprietary names even though specific reference to this fact is not always made in the text. Therfore, the appearance of a name without designation as proprietary is not to be construed as a representation by the publisher that it is in the public domain.
All rights, including the rights of publication, distribution and sales, as well as the right to translation, are reserved. No part of this work covered by the copyrights hereon may be reproduced or copied in any form or by any means − graphic, electronic or mechanical including photocopying, recording, taping, or information and retrieval systems − without written permission ot the publishers.

© 1981 Georg Thieme Verlag, Herdweg 63, D-7000 Stuttgart 1, FRG
Typesetting by Tutte Druckerei GmbH, D-8391 Salzweg, on Lino-VIP
Printed in West Germany by Aumüller, D-8400 Regensburg

ISBN 3-13-612601-7

5  4  3  2  1  0

# Foreword by the Translator

This atlas presents in a precise and concise form the most important and salient aspects of clinical ophthalmology. Professor Hollwich has collected these pictures over the last two decades when he was Professor and Chairman of the Department of Ophthalmology at the University of Muenster. The pictures are of such high quality that they present the best facsimile of true life conditions we can expect.

The atlas is put together in such a way that it should serve as a quick reference for any medical student, intern, family practitioner, or other nonophthalmic physician. It allows a quick diagnosis of the most frequent ocular anomalies and diseases.

The text is kept extremely short on purpose. This hand atlas should not replace any textbook, but should serve as a quick illustrative guide for the recognition of ocular disorders.

Iowa City, Iowa, Spring of 1981.                    F. C. Blodi, M. D.

# Preface

Ophthalmology is like no other specialty in medicine, a science where most pathologic changes can be visualized. With the help of optical instruments, we are able to examine and photograph nearly every part of the eye. Even the most careful description of a pathologic process remains incomplete without a photo to document it.

An atlas, i. e. a collection of pictures, has always been an integral part in the teaching of medicine, especially of ophthalmology, and even for the practising ophthalmologist or for a physician in another specialty, an atlas is an excellent means to get a quick information and a pictorial explanation of ocular changes.

The collection of pictures in this pocket book represents typical disease processes as they are seen in the daily practice. It gives an overview of ophthalmology illustrating in colored photos the most common anomalies and diseases of the anterior segment and of the fundus.

The collection was enlarged by seven colored photographs of juvenile macular degenerations which Professor J. François of Ghent put at our disposal. I would like to thank here also my long-time collaborator at the University Eye Clinic in Muenster, Dr. B. Verbeck.

My special gratitude goes to Dr. med. h. c. G. Hauff for stimulating me to produce this pocket atlas and for his and his collaborators' help in publishing it.

Munich, Summer of 1980.                                  F. HOLLWICH

# Contents

# 1. Lids

The lids protect the eyeball and may show numerous congenital anomalies and pathologic changes. These may affect the lids alone or may occur in connection with systemic diseases.

The anomalies and pathologic changes are manifest in many forms. They may affect the skin of the lids, the tarsus, the striated and smooth musculature of the lid, the remarkably well-developed blood and lymph vessels, as well as the numerous nerves, such as the trigeminal, the oculomotor and the facial nerves, which are cranial nerves, and the sympathetic nerve, which is part of the autonomic nervous system. The lids are a conspicuous part of the face and therefore even small or minute pathologic changes will be noticed early. A survey of the numerous congenital anomalies and various diseases and injuries of the lids is of interest not only for ophthalmologists and dermatologists but also for family practitioners and for many other specialists.

We have tried in the following series of illustrations to present the topic according to a uniform anatomical and physiologic viewpoint.

The chapter begins with a discussion on the most frequent inflammations and diseases of the skin and glands of the lid, which represent a major part of all lid diseases. The conditions include infections and inflammations of the skin, allergic reactions and lid edema of various etiology, eczema and inflammations of the lid glands, as well as injuries of the lids including those involving the ethmoidal cells. Injuries of the lids involving the lacrimal system will be discussed later.

Other illustrations depict congenital anomalies and abnormal positions of the lids (ptosis). Their surgical correction will be alluded to. This part also includes congenital and acquired disturbances of lid motions, which may occur as an isolated phenomenon or involve several muscles affecting opening and closing of the lids. These disturbances may involve not only the striated muscles (orbicularis and levator), but also the smooth muscles (superior and inferior Mueller muscles). Other disturbances of lid motility involve also movements of the eyeball.

Numerous illustrations depict tumors of the lids. Among the congenital tumefactions are dermoid, nevus, hemangioma and lymphangioma, lipoma and neurofibroma. Other illustrations show acquired cysts and tumors (xanthelasma, milia, retention cyst, cutaneous horn and verruca vulgaris), as well as malignant lesions, such as basal cell carcinoma and rhabdomyosarcoma.

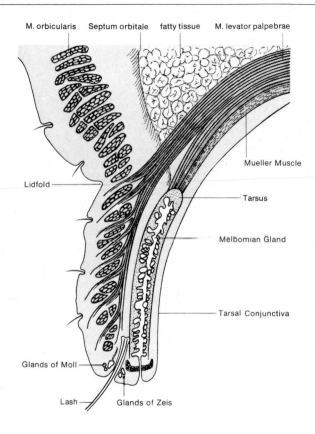

M. orbicularis   Septum orbitale   fatty tissue   M. levator palpebrae

Mueller Muscle

Lidfold

Tarsus

Melbomian Gland

Tarsal Conjunctiva

Glands of Moll

Lash   Glands of Zeis

Fig 1-1   Cross section through the upper lid (schematic). The secretion of the sebaceous glands (meibomian glands and glands of Zeis) covers the palpebral margin so that the tears will normally not run over the cheek. The glands of Moll are modified sweat glands.
The orbicularis muscle, which closes the lids, and the levator and Mueller muscles, which open the lids, are schematically drawn. The levator muscle inserts into the skin, the tarsus and the orbicularis muscle. Mueller's muscle also inserts into the upper margin of the tarsus (*Hollwich, F*.: Augenheilkunde, 9th ed. Stuttgart: Thieme 1979).

Fig 1-2   Coloboma of the right upper lid in the Goldenhar syndrome which involves the eye and the ear. The external part of the ear is small and there is a whorl deformity of the right brow. There is an anomalous position of the teeth (5-year-old boy).

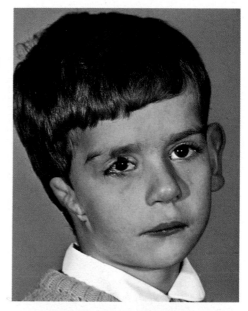

Fig 1-3   Hemiatrophy of the face on the left side with anophthalmos and small left ala of the nose. There is a severe deformity of the external portion of the ear and circumscribed scleroderma (5-week-old girl).

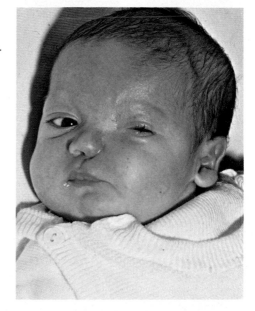

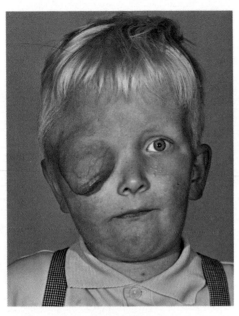

Fig 1-4   Hypertrophy of the right side of the face with elephantiasis of the right upper lid in neurofibromatosis (von *Recklinghausen* disease). Soft, noninflammatory thickening of the right upper lid which hangs like a thick fold over the right cheek. The right orbit is enlarged and the right globe lies deep in the orbit (5-year-old boy).

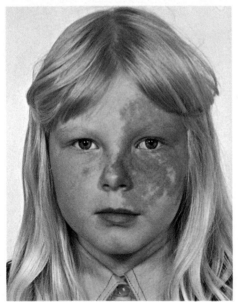

Fig 1-5   Nevus flammeus on the left side of the face. The left globe is enlarged and the intraocular pressure is increased (Sturge-Weber syndrome). The skin in the involved area has a red-violet color which blanches on pressure. The lesion is strictly unilateral and follows the distribution of the trigeminal nerve. There is hemangioma of the conjunctiva and the choroid. The palpebral fissure on the left is widened and there is also a hemangiomatous change of the episclera (8-year-old girl).

Fig 1-6  Acute measles exanthema. This begins in the face and the lesions are first small, round or oval, but coalesce later. They are dark red and slightly elevated over the skin. They merge to form large plaques separated by small unaffected skin areas. The acute stage begins with an inflammation of the nose, the pharynx, the trachea and the bronchi, usually after high fever. This is followed by conjunctivitis and photophobia (4-year-old girl).

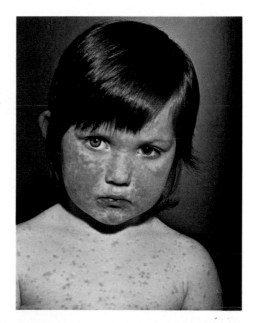

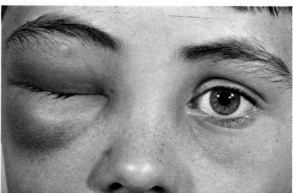

Fig 1-7  Lid edema after an insect bite. The right upper lid had been stung below the brow. A serous fluid is exuded due to an allergic reaction. Because of gravity the fluid may also invade the lower lid. Pseudoptosis (8-year-old boy).

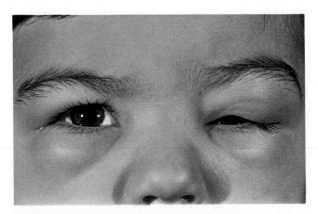

Fig 1-8   Acute bilateral lid edema. The face is pale and pasty due to an allergic reaction to an intestinal worm infection (oxyuriasis). Eosinophilia of the blood (3-year-old girl).

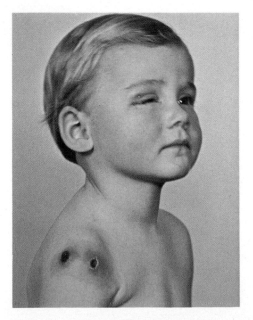

Fig 1-9   Vaccinia of the lids 2 weeks after a vaccination. This is a self-infection and occurred on the same side as the vaccination (1-year-old girl).

Fig 1-10 Impetigo contagiosa with lid involvement. This infection, caused by streptococci, is an acute skin eruption involving the face. There are intraepidermal pustules, vesicles and yellow-gray crusts with yellow borders and hemorrhages. Black crusts can be seen at the inner canthus, on the nose and on the front (13-year-old boy).

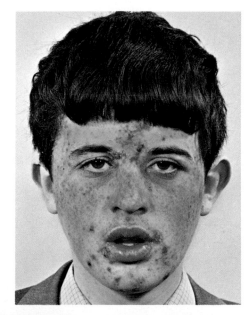

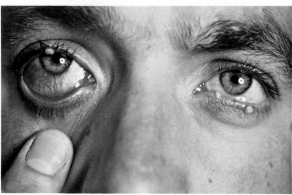

Fig 1-11 Molluscum contagiosum. White-yellow, pearly nodules of varying size and with a central depression lie on both upper and lower lids. They contain keratinized epithelial cells with inclusion bodies. This is a benign viral infection usually involving the skin of the face and of the lids (23-year-old man).

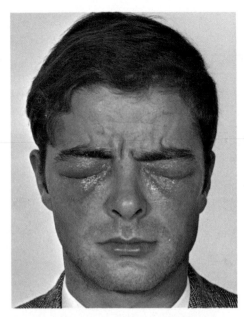

Fig 1-12   Acute contact dermatitis of the lids due to an allergy to chloramphenicol. There is marked erythema and edema with the formation of vesicles involving the epidermis of the lids. After a short time these vesicles burst leaving a weeping surface. There is photophobia and blepharospasm (25-year-old man).

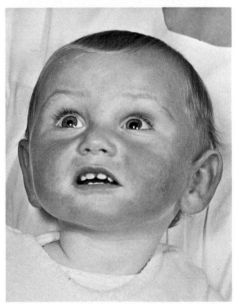

Fig 1-13   Contact dermatitis of the face because the patient was sensitive to atropine. There is erythema and hyperemia of the facial skin including the ears. This occurred after the administration of one drop of 1% atropine before a refraction (13-month-old girl).

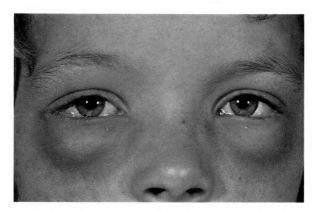

Fig 1-14    Allergic edema of the lids in hay fever. There is mild conjunctival injection and bilateral chemosis. Tissue fluid accumulates in the lower lids (5-year-old boy).

Fig 1-15    Emphysema of the lids. There is marked swelling of the left upper and lower lids after an injury to the ethmoidal cells 3 days earlier. Because of the injury to the sinuses, air was pressed into the lids when the pressure in the nose increased (blowing the nose, sneezing). Crepitus on palpation (29-year-old man).

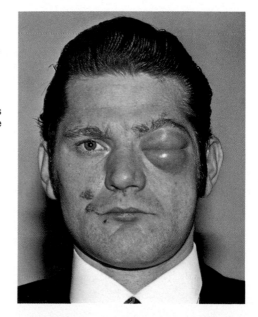

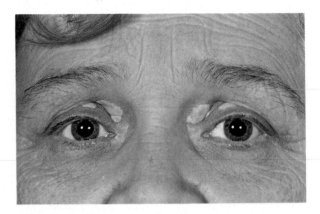

Fig 1-16   Xanthelasma. Symmetrical lipid deposits into the skin of the lids at the inner canthus. Most frequently seen in women at menopause. Occasionally it may indicate diabetes mellitus, metabolic disturbances or vascular diseases of the heart or of the extremities (53-year-old woman).

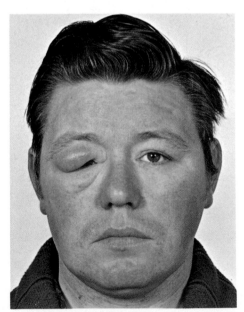

Fig 1-17   Familial blepharochalasis. This becomes apparent in puberty and is characterized by an intermittent edema of the upper lids. Here the right lid is more affected than the left one. There is no pain during the attack and the edema disappears again after 1-2 days (40-year-old man).

Fig 1-18   Ascher syndrome. Familial juvenile blepharochalasis with anomaly of the upper lip (there is a hair-free zone immediately above the vermilion border) combined with a goiter. The condition is here more pronounced on the right than on the left side (14-year-old boy).

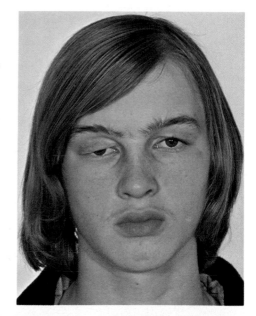

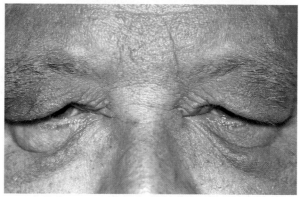

Fig 1-19   Presenile dermatochalasis. A loose skin fold of the upper lid hangs like a curtain over the palpebral margin reaching the lower lid. There is some bulging of the lower lid ("bags"). The palpebral fissure is closed except for a small slitlike opening nasally (55-year-old man).

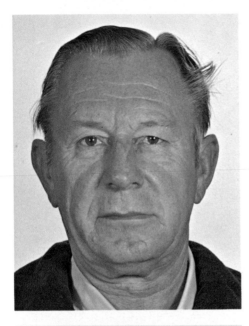

Fig 1-20   Bilateral senile dermatochalasis. The skin of the upper lids is thin and loose hanging like a fold over the palpebral margin (64-year-old man).

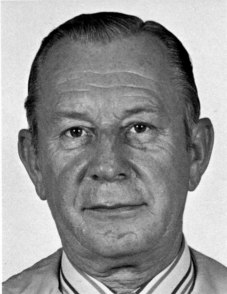

Fig 1-21   Same patient as in Figure 1-20. Several months after a blepharoplasty (Hollwich, F. and Illig, K. M.: Klin. Monatsbl. Augenheilkd. 166:255, 1975).

Fig 1-22  "Bags" of the lower lids. Because of dehiscence and loosening of the orbital septum, the orbital fat prolapses like a hernia into the subcutaneous tissue. This usually occurs in middle age or senescence (64-year-old man).

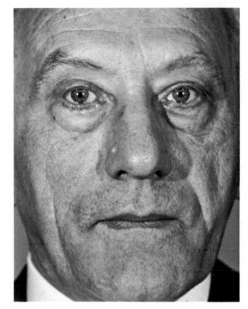

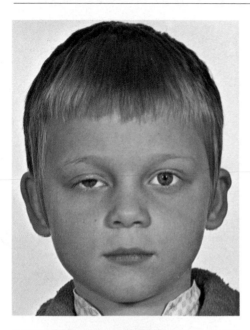

Fig 1-23   Congenital ptosis on the right. The upper lid droops to the level of the pupillary center (6-year-old boy).

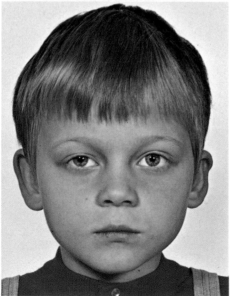

Fig 1-24   Same patient as in Figure 1-23 six weeks after a ptosis operation. The palpebral fissures are now equal in both eyes (6-year-old boy).

Fig 1-25 Congenital ptosis on the sight. The droopy upper lid covers the upper part of the pupil (29-year-old woman).

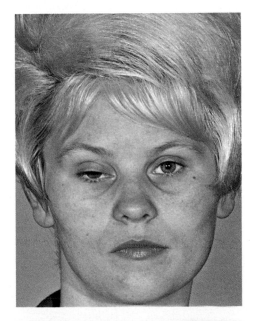

Fig 1-26 Same patient as In Figure 1-25 eight weeks after a ptosis operation with resection and advancement of the levator muscle. The palpebral fissures are now equal on both sides and the right pupil is no longer covered (29-year-old woman).

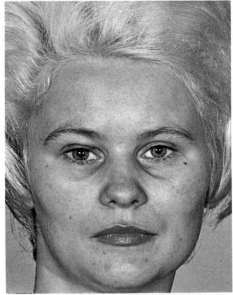

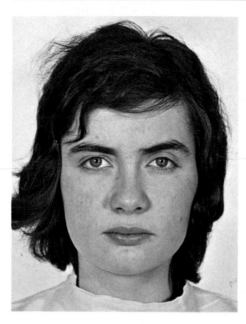

Fig 1-27   Horner's syndrome on the left. Ptosis, miosis and enophthalmos. The palpebral fissure on the left is smaller than on the right and the left pupil is constricted. There is a weakness of the smooth Mueller's muscle, the dilator of the pupil and the orbitalis muscle because of a congenital paresis of the sympathetic nerve on that side (20-year-old woman).

Fig 1-28   Paralytic ptosis with complete oculomotor paresis on the right side. The paretic upper lid cannot be voluntarily elevated (46-year-old woman).

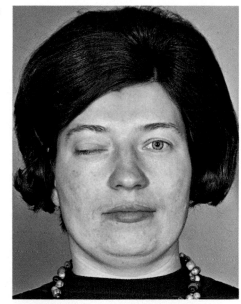

Fig 1-29   Same patient as in Figure 1-28 with the upper lid elevated. The globe is turned out because the external rectus (innervated by the sixth nerve) is still functioning. There is slight protrusion of the globe because the normal tonic traction of the extraocular muscles innervated by the oculomotor nerve (superior, inferior, medial rectus and inferior oblique) is lacking. If the patient tries to look down the eye will show an inward torsion. This is due to the action of the superior oblique muscle (innervated by the trochlear nerve). The pupil is widely dilated and reacts slowly to light and with convergence: incomplete internal and complete external oculomotor paresis (46-year-old woman).

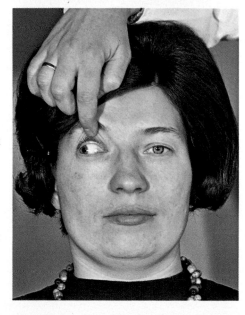

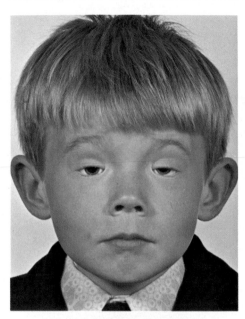

Fig 1-30   Ptosis with Waardenburg syndrome. Combination of epicanthus, congenital ptosis and shortened palpebral fissure (blepharophimosis). Occasionally strabismus. Compensatory elevation of the lid by using the frontalis muscle. Hereditary disturbance of the position of the lid (5-year-old boy).

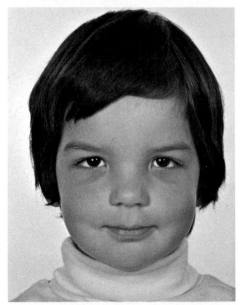

Fig 1-31   Epicanthus, a congenital anomaly, in a small child. The skin fold over the upper lid is longer than normal and covers the inner canthus as well as the semilunar fold and the caruncle. This can mimic strabismus. The condition improves when the root of the nose grows and becomes more elevated (5-year-old boy).

Fig 1-32  Congenital ptosis with synkinesis of the right upper lid and the jaw (jaw-winking phenomenon of Marcus-Gunn). The right upper lid is ptotic and there is narrowing of the palpebral fissure, temporally more than nasally (10-year-old boy).

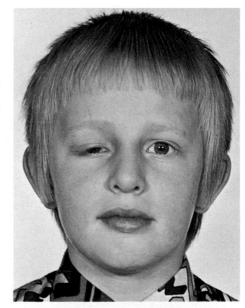

Fig 1-33  With movements of the jaw (chewing or lateral movements) there is an abrupt reflex elevation of the right upper lid. The cause is probably an aberrant innervation with cross signals between the facial, trigeminal and oculomotor nerves (10-year-old boy).

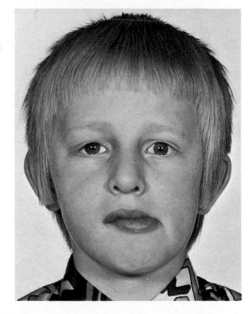

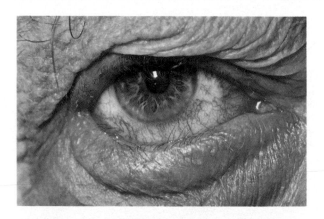

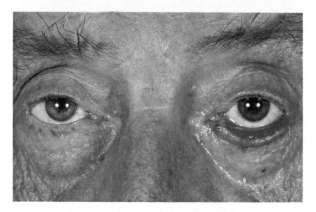

Fig 1-34   Senile spastic entropion. There is a contracture of the lower part of the orbicularis muscle. The palpebral margin has turned inward. The lashes are pointing toward the eyeball and scratch bulbar conjunctiva and cornea (pseudotrichiasis). Chronic conjunctivitis. Danger of developing a corneal erosion or ulcer (73-year-old man).

Fig 1-35   Senile ectropion. The left lower lid is loose and turned outward. The palpebral margin has become blunt and the exposed conjunctiva is thickened and chronically inflamed. The lower punctum is turned away from the conjunctival sac and therefore the tears run down the cheek (epiphora). There is a tendency to wipe the lower lid frequently which aggravates the entropion and establishes a vicious cycle (74-year-old man).

Fig 1-36  Bilateral senile ectropion. The lower lids are loose and turned outward. The palpebral margins are blunt and the exposed tarsal conjunctiva is thickened and chronically inflamed. There is epiphora aggravated by wiping the lids (70-year-old man).

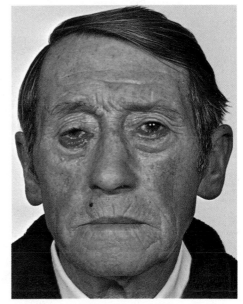

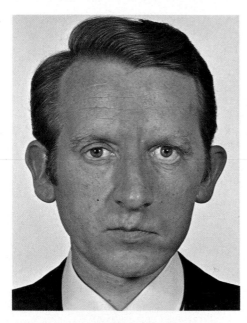

Fig 1-37  Paralytic ectropion with palsy of the left peripheral facial nerve. All three branches are affected: the front (smoothened skin folds), the eye (lagophthalmos) and the mouth (smoothened nasolabial fold and drooping mouth on the left side) (43-year-old man).

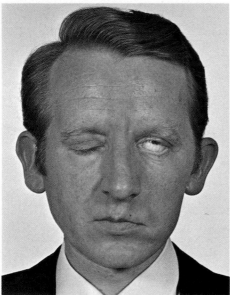

Fig 1-38  Lagophthalmos on the left side with paresis of the facial nerve (same patient as in Figure 1-37). Bell's phenomenon (on attempted lid closure the eye rolls upward). This protects the corneal epithelium from drying out during sleep. Only a small lower segment of the cornea is usually exposed.

Fig 1-39  Cicatricial ectropion after injury. A keloid-like scar pulls the lower lid downward and outward. The scar is adherent to the bony orbital margin. There is chronic irritation of the tarsal conjunctiva, with epiphora because the lower punctum is turned away from the conjunctival sac. The palpebral margin is blunt (38-year-old man).

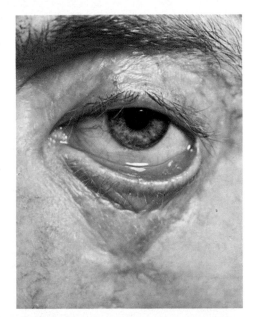

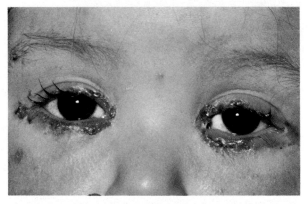

Fig 1-40  Ulcerous blepharitis. Yellowish crusts and deposits lie between the matted lashes. There is a purulent, thick secretion on the thickened palpebral margins. Staphylococcal infection (4-year-old girl).

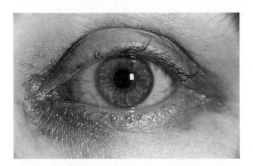

Fig 1-41   Angular blepharitis. Infection with diplobacillus involving the margin between skin and mucous membrane. The palpebral margin, especially of the canthal areas, is involved. Because of the action of proteolytic enzymes produced by the diplobacilli, the affected areas have a violet color. This extends into the upper and lower lid (25-year-old man).

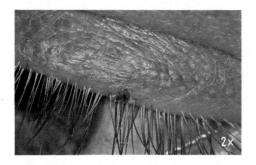

Fig 1-42   Phthiriasis of the lashes. The eggs of pubic lice are deposited at the base of the lashes and appear as brown-black nodules (24-year-old man).

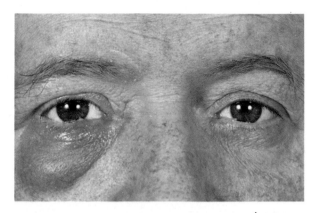

Fig 1-43   Internal hordeolum of the right lower lid. This is an acute inflammation of the meibomian gland. A pus-filled vesicle can be seen in the center of the lid margin at the opening of an excretory duct of a meibomian gland. There is lid edema with circumscribed bulging of the skin of the lower lid. The regional lymph nodes in front of the ear and at the jaw are tender and swollen (45-year-old man):

Fig 1-44   External hordeolum. Acute inflammation of a sebaceous Zeis gland at the external canthus of the upper lid. Spontaneous perforation of the hordeolum at the follicle of a lash (12-year-old boy).

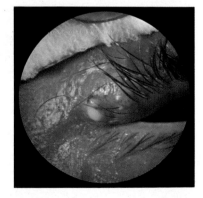

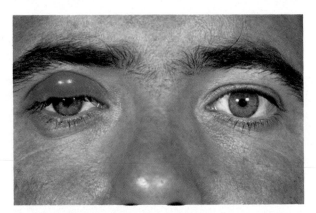

Fig 1-45 Chalazion. Painless, noninfectious, tumefaction in the middle of the right upper lid. Chronic occlusion of the excretory ducts of meibomian glands (28-year-old man).

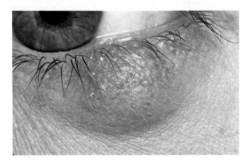

Fig 1-46 Chalazion. Chronic obstruction of the meibomian gland. Nontender and painless. There is a hard tumefaction in the middle of the lid (30-year-old woman).

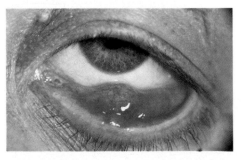

Fig 1-47 When the lower lid is pulled downward an indolent nodule is seen on the inner aspect of the lower lid. It corresponds to one of the meibomian glands in the tarsus. The nodule extends toward the lid margin (49-year-old woman).

Fig 1-48   Subperiosteal abscess. Fluctuating tumefaction of the left upper lid with chemosis. The globe is pushed forward and downward. The patient had an elevated temperature (39 °C). The periost was slit at the temporal orbital margin and a drain inserted under local anesthesia. Uneventful healing (4-week-old boy).

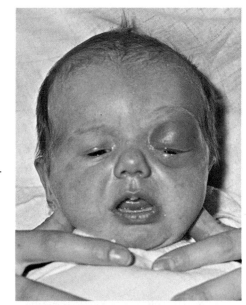

Fig 1-49   Dermoid cyst of the left upper lid and brow. Spherical, elastic protrusion at the temporal upper area. Congenital displacement of epidermis. Usually located close to a bone suture. The skin over the cyst is freely movable. Differential diagnosis: meningocele (1-year-old boy).

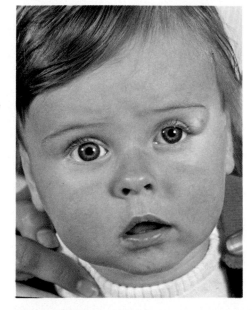

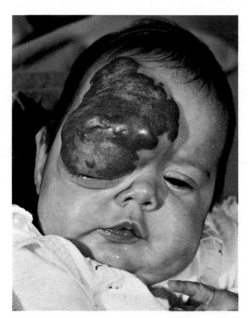

Fig 1-50 Hemangioma of the right side of the face. Extensive, partly cavernous hemangioma involving the right upper lid and the frontal area. The child was born 8 weeks prematurely and spent 1 week in an incubator. The tumor started as a pinpoint-like lesion and was treated with a strontium applicator on the 7th and 18th days of life. After that rapid growth occured (4½-month-old girl).

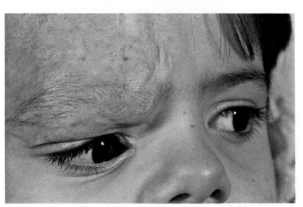

Fig 1-51 Same child as in Figure 1-50 five years later. The hemangioma decreased in size with the application of pressure bandages. There is now esotropia and hypotropia of the right eye with amblyopia. With occlusion therapy to the left eye, visual acuity in the right increased to 0,6 (5-year-old girl).

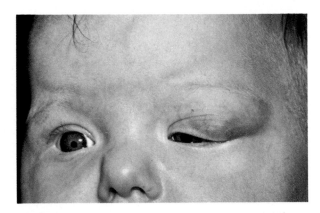

Fig 1-52    Hemangioma of the left upper lid. Bluish red, soft tumefaction at the outer canthus. When the child cries the tumor increases in size because of increased blood flow (6-month-old girl).

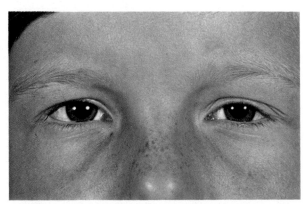

Fig 1-53    Same child as in Figure 1-52 seven years later. Spontaneous regression of the hemangioma with cosmetically acceptable result (7$\frac{1}{2}$-year-old girl).

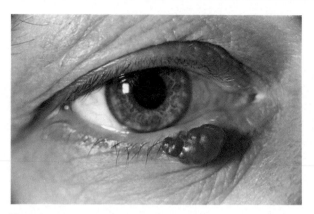

Fig 1-54   Hemangioma. Strawberry-like, blue red tumefaction with nodular surface. Congenital cavernous hemangioma with the stalk attached to the lower lid (48-year-old woman).

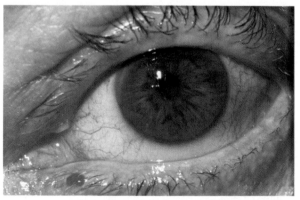

Fig 1-55   Senile hemangioma. Pinpoint-sized bright red nodule on the left lower lid below the lacrimal punctum (77-year-old woman).

Fig 1-56   Pseudoptosis on the right. Elephantiasis of the upper lid in neurofibromatosis (von Recklinghausen disease). Soft, noninflammatory, diffuse thickening of the temporal part of the right upper lid. Café-au-lait spots at the root of the nose, left frontal area, eyebrows, cheeks and back (3-year-old girl).

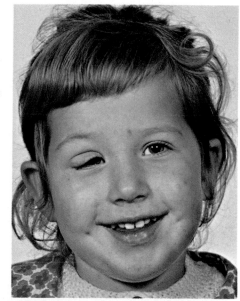

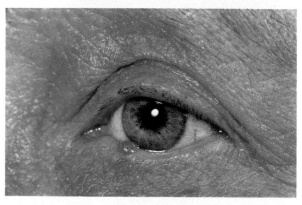

Fig 1-57   Papilloma of the left lower lid. In the middle of the palpebral margin above the row of lashes an indolent, small, firm nodule (62-year-old man).

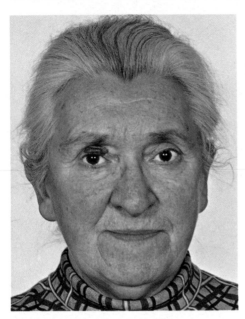

Fig 1-58   Pigmented hairy nevus. The flat, benign, partly hairy pigmentation extends over two-thirds of the right, slightly thickened upper lid (68-year-old woman).

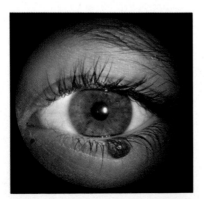

Fig 1-59   Keratinized papilloma. In the middle of the left lower lid is a pea-sized, firm, brown-yellow nodule with an irregular surface (8-year-old girl).

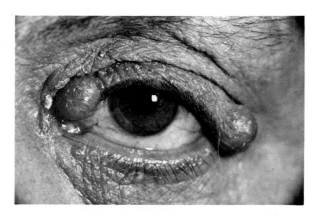

Fig 1-60  Retention cyst of a Moll gland. Cysts derived from these sweat glands hang from the palpebral canthi. They contain a watery, transparent fluid (67-year-old woman).

Fig 1-61  Verruca in the middle of the left upper lid. Small, pale tumor with slightly irregular surface (5-year-old girl).

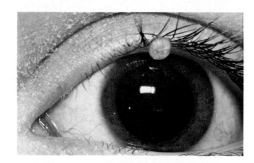

Fig 1-62  Keratoacanthoma. Hemispherical, bean-sized, indolent nodule in the middle of the left lower lid (63-year-old man).

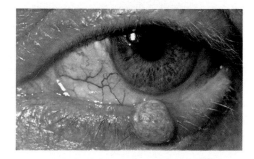

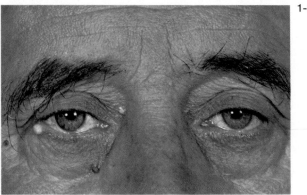

1-63

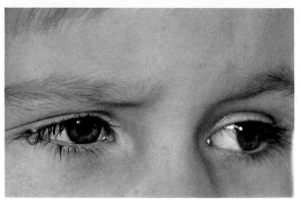

1-64

Fig 1-63   Retention cyst of the right lower lid. Small, yellowish nodule at the external canthus and in the right upper lid above the internal canthus (62-year-old man).

Fig 1-64   Warts of the right upper and lower lid. Small, yellow-white tumefactions with irregular surface on the lower lid and close to the external canthus. On the upper lid a small "kissing" wart (5-year-old boy).

1-65

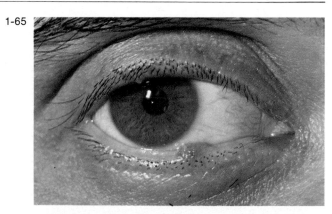

1-66

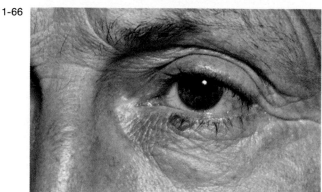

Fig 1-65  Tumor in the middle of the right lower lid. Small, red-yellow nodule with smooth surface at the palpebral margin in the central third of the lower lid. Histologic examination: lipoma (23-year-old man).

Fig 1-66  Carcinoma. Small, elevated tumor with a hard margin and depressed central area in the middle of the left lower lid. Histologic examination indicated basal cell carcinoma (60-year-old man).

1-67

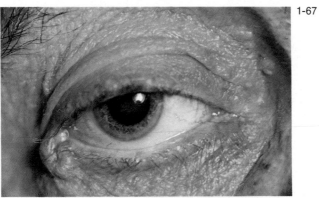

1-68

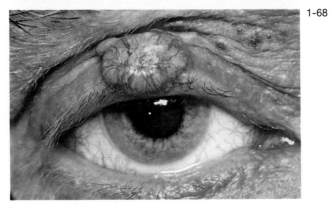

Fig 1-67   Basal cell carcinoma of the right external canthus. Typical elevated margin with a pearly surface. The center of the tumor is depressed (74-year-old man).

Fig 1-68   Basal cell carcinoma. A bean-sized vascularized tumor with elevated margins in the center of the right upper lid. Beginning necrosis in the center (69-year-old man).

1-69

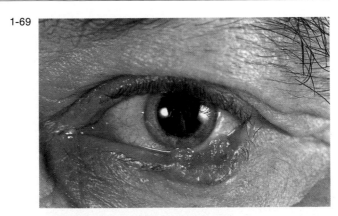

1-70

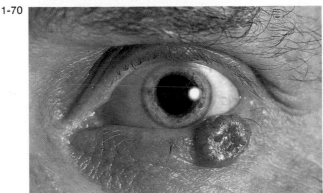

Fig 1-69   Basal cell carcinoma. Flat, plaquelike tumor of the lower lid. In some areas the normal palpebral margin is destroyed and thickened by tumor infiltration. The margins are slightly elevated, the center is ulcerated and bleeding. Histologic examination indicated basal cell carcinoma (68-year-old man).

Fig 1-70   Basal cell carcinoma of the left lower lid margin. Elevated, pearly margins with depressed hemorrhagic center (52-year-old man).

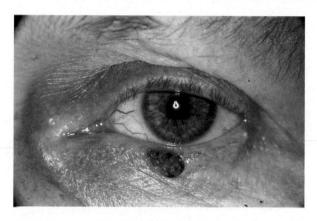

Fig 1-71    Nevus. Pigmented, slightly elevated tumor in the center of the left lower lid (57-year-old woman).

# 2. Lacrimal System

The lacrimal system consists of a tear-producing (lacrimal gland) and tear-conducting part (canaliculi, lacrimal sac, nasolacrimal duct).

The outflow of tears is facilitated by an active pump. Fibers of the lacrimal part of the orbicularis muscle (Horner's muscle) contract the puncta and the canaliculi. Synchronous with lid closure there is a lateral movement of the lids, inward torsion of the palpebral margins, dipping of the puncta into the lacrimal lake and alternating opening and closing of the canaliculi. The flow of tears is also facilitated by suction from the nose. Each olincing on th ot only a wetting of the cornea, but also a "biologic irrigation" of the conjunctival sac cleansing it from dust and microorganisms.

There are a variety of diseases of the lacrimal system. The following illustrations show anomalies of the puncta and a previously popular operation, slitting of the canaliculus (one-snip operation), acute and chronic dacryoadenitis and dacryocystitis as well as the effects of a surgical dacryocystorhinostomy (Kaleff-Hollwich modification of the Toti procedure).

Another picture illustrates the painless and bloodless probing of a congenital stenosis of the nasolacrimal duct. Such probing does not usually lead to any complications. Before the procedure, a local anesthetic solution, warmed to body temperature to avoid local, painful irritation, should be dropped into the conjunctival sac. It is advisable to irrigate first with a vasoconstrictor to shrink the mucous membrane of the lacrimal sac and constrict the surrounding blood vessels. This will lead to a smoothening of the mucosal folds so that the probe will not be caught in a blind pocket. A false route can thus be avoided and the probe can be pushed into the nasolacrimal duct and into the nose.

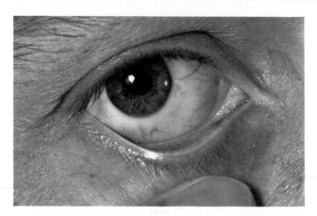

Fig 2-1   Congenital anomaly: double lower punctum in the right eye. On irrigation both puncta connected with the canaliculus (34-year-old woman).

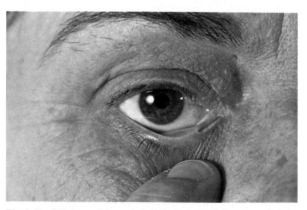

Fig 2-2   Slitting of lower punctum (one-snip operation). This method is usually not successful, but was previously used in older patients for epiphora. It is unsuccessful because cutting the sphincter-like annular musculature of the punctum weakens the active pump and suction mechanism of the tear flow. In addition, the punctum may turn away from the bulbar conjunctiva or a secondary, cicatricial dacryostenosis may develop aggravating the condition instead of improving it (56-year-old woman).

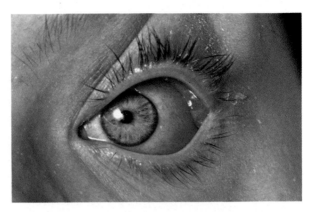

Fig 2-3   Abscess of the lacrimal gland on the left. Unilateral tender swelling of the upper lid with conjunctival injection and chemosis. When the upper lid is elevated the inflamed and swollen palpebral part of the lacrimal gland is visible. The preauricular lymph nodes are swollen (13-year-old girl).

Fig 2-4   Abscess of the lacrimal sac. Fluctuating, inflammatory swelling in the area of the fossa lacrimalis. The preauricular and submandibular lymph nodes are swollen. The patient had an elevated temperature. Etiology: damage to the mucosal membrane of the nasolacrimal duct with subsequent infection after a probing, which was not preceded by irrigation with a vasoconstrictor (2$^1/_2$-month-old boy).

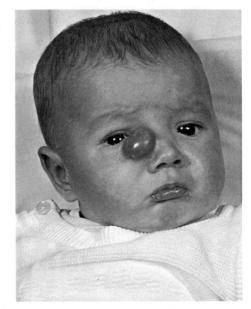

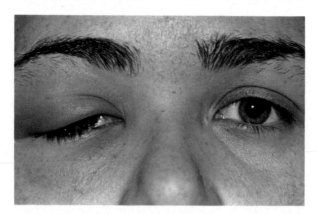

Fig 2-5   Acute dacryoadenitis. Pressure sensitive, inflammatory swelling of the lacrimal gland which lies at the upper outer aspect of the orbit. Inflammatory pseudoptosis. Due to the swelling the palpebral margin of the upper lid acquires an S-shape (20-year-old woman).

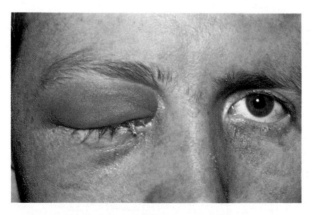

Fig 2-6   Orbital abscess (early stage). A drinking straw penetrated deep into the orbit. There is now an inflammatory swelling of the upper and to a lesser degree of the lower lid. Purulent cellulitis. Exophthalmos and marked decrease in ocular motility. At the inner canthus the chemotic conjunctiva is prolapsed (25-year-old man).

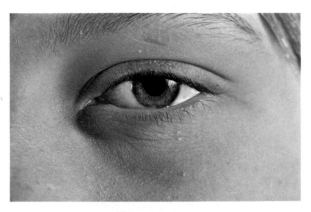

Fig 2-7   Dacryocystitis on the left. Beneath the punctum is a spherical fluctuating swelling with chemosis of the adjacent conjunctiva (13-year-old boy).

Fig 2-8   Probing of the nasolacrimal duct in an infant. A local anesthetic is dropped into the conjunctival sac and the lacrimal system is irrigated with a vasoconstrictor to decrease the swelling of the mucous membrane in the lacrimal sac. The probing can be performed without pain and without complications (1$\frac{1}{2}$-year-old girl).

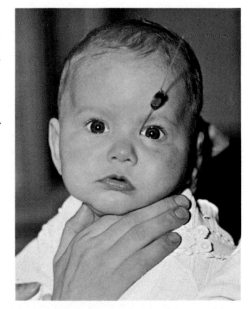

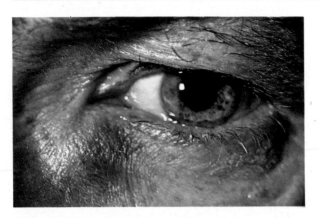

Fig 2 9   Dacryocystitis with chronic dacryostenosis. There is a hemispherical, subcutaneous, fluctuating mass in the area of the lacrimal sac. (25-year-old man).

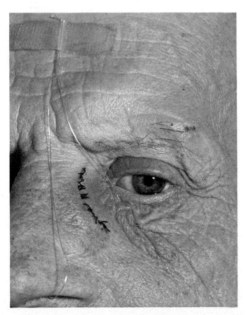

Fig 2-10   Three days earlier this patient had had a dacryocystorhinostomy (Kaleff-Hollwich method), performed because of complete dacryostenosis. Anylon thread is used as a stent and will remain for 10-14 days (Hollwich, F.: Klin. Monatsbl. Augenheilkd. 170:633, 1977) (67-year-old man).

# 3. Conjunctiva

The conjunctiva is a mucous membrane which lies as a thin and transparent layer loosely over the eyeball, but is firmly adherent to the inside of the lids. The epithelial layer contains goblet cells which secrete mucin and combat external injurious agents. The same is achieved by the lysozyme, a bacteriostatic agent which is contained in the tear fluid. The conjunctiva rarely shows degenerative changes, but is frequently exposed to trauma and allergic and infectious insult.

The following microorganisms are most frequently the cause of an infectious conjunctivitis:
- Cocci (e. g., staphylococci, streptococci, pneumococci)
- Bacteria (e. g., diplobacillus Morax-Axenfeld, diplobacillus Koch-Weeks, *Pseudomonas aeruginosa, corynebacterium diphtheriae*)
- A virus (e. g., APC virus type 8, herpes hominis virus type 1)
  Clamydia agents (TRIC agents as a cause of trachoma and neonatal inclusion conjunctivitis)
- Fungi (e. g., *Candida albicans*)
- Parasites (e. g., *Onchocerca volvolus*)

Like any other mucous membrane the conjunctiva reacts to noxious agents with the development of an acute infection which may involve all three parts of this organ (bulbar, tarsal and fornix). The secretion may be watery, mucinous or purulent.

The following illustrations depict pinguecula and pterygium, allergic conjunctivitis, vernal catarrh and acute conjunctivitis. These are followed with pictures of other conjunctival diseases, hemorrhages into the conjunctiva after a trauma, as well as blepharoconjunctivitis. Epidemic keratoconjunctivitis will be discussed in detail illustrating its clinical picture and course. Finally, a few rare conjunctival diseases will be illustrated: conjunctival phlyctenule, squamous cell carcinoma, nevus and melanoma of the conjunctiva.

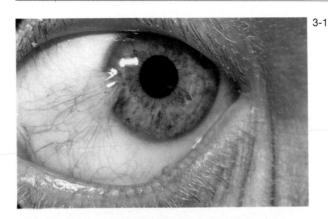

3-1

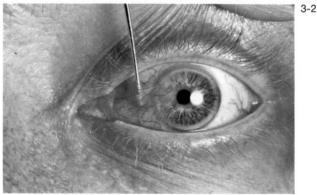

3-2

Fig 3-1   Pterygium. Triangular, thin, transparent conjunctival fold in the palpebral fissure. Its head is yellow, avascular and points toward the corneal center. The body of the pterygium extends to the semilunar fold (32-year-old man).

Fig 3-2   Cicatricial pterygium. Differential diagnosis: the margins of the cicatricial pterygium cannot be elevated with a probe or a forceps. This is in contrast to true pterygium. In the cicatricial type the conjunctival folds are irregular, thickened and vascularized. This type does not show a tendency to progress toward the cornea. Characteristics: white, adherent to the site of corneal injury, with no avascular head. Cause: burn, chemical injury. In this case there was injury at the limbus (65-year-old man).

3-3

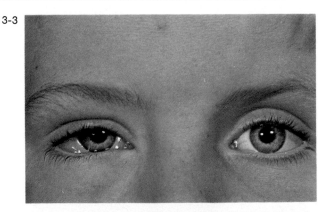

3-4

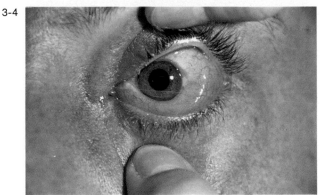

Fig 3-3   Allergic conjunctivitis. Chemosis, i. e., elevation of the bulbar conjunctiva from the sclera by an exudation of fluid. The allergic reaction was
here produced by blooming grass. Such a conjunctivitis occurs also with
hay fever (10-year-old boy).

Fig 3-4   Allergic conjunctivitis. Marked exudation of fluid under the bulbar
conjunctiva which shows a bulbous detachment. The allergy was due to
pollen (22-year-old man).

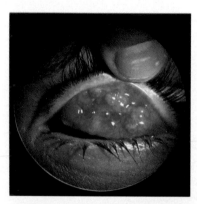

Fig 3-5   Vernal catarrh. Cobble-stone-like proliferations of the tarsal conjunctiva (everted upper lid) (12-year-old boy).

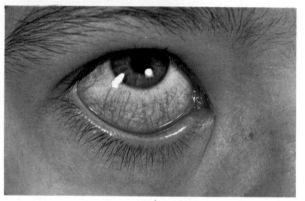

Fig 3-6   Acute conjunctivitis. Hyperemia and chemosis of all three segments of the conjunctiva (bulbar, fornix and tarsal). The vermillion-red conjunctival vessels can be moved against the sclera. There is an increased watery and mucous secretion. The cause may be mechanical, chemical-physical, bacterial or viral (12-year-old girl).

3-7

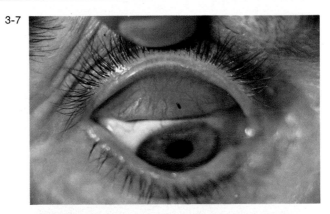

3-8

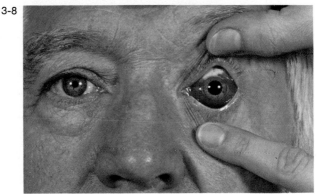

Fig 3-7   Subtarsal foreign body. Broken off insect wing. On everting the upper lid the foreign body shifted from the subtarsal sulcus downward (40-year-old woman).

Fig 3-8   Subconjunctival hemorrhage on the left. Injury with the tip of a palm leaf (60-year-old man).

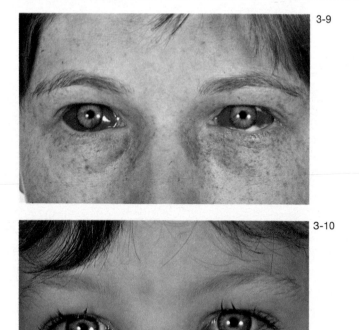

Fig 3-9   Bilateral subconjunctival hemorrhages. Prolonged Valsalva maneuver during delivery (27-year-old woman).

Fig 3-10   Purulent blepharoconjunctivitis. Inflammatory hyperemia and chemosis of the conjunctiva. Serous and purulent secretion at the inner canthus. The lids stick together in the morning because of the dried, purulent secretion. The smear shows pneumococci (4-year-old girl).

Fig 3-11   Bilateral angular blepharoconjunctivitis. Pale pink discoloration of the canthus. White stringy secretion. Only minimal conjunctival injection. Smear showed diplobacillus Morax-Axenfeld; treatment with antibiotics (2-year-old boy).

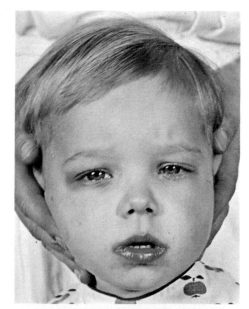

Fig 3-12   Epidemic keratoconjunctivitis. Highly Infectious viral disease produced by type 8 of the adenopharyngoconjunctival virus group (APC). After an incubation period of 8 days there is unilateral pseudoptosis, swelling and redness of the caruncle and semilunar fold with follicles in the fornix. Conjunctival hemorrhages appear because the vessel walls are damaged by the virus. Swelling of the preauricular and submandibular lymph nodes. Beginning redness of the semilunar fold on the left. In previous epidemics up to 50% of the patients had corneal involvement (superficial keratitis) (30-year-old man).

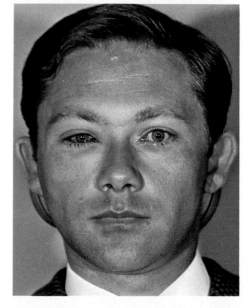

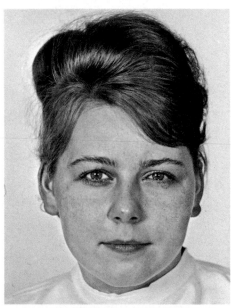

Fig 3-13   Epidemic keratoconjunctivitis. In the early stage there was a unilateral involvement of the left eye with photophobia and foreign body sensation. Pseudoptosis. The right eye is still white. Influenza-like general symptoms with a mild fever. The disease is highly contagious and may affect whole families, occupants of one house or patients of one clinic (transmission by tonometry!) (21-year-old woman).

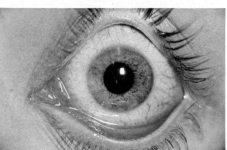

Fig 3-14   Epidemic keratoconjunctivitis. The left eye in higher magnification (same patient as in Figure 3-13). Redness and swelling of the caruncle and semilunar fold as well as the fornix. Minimal secretion.

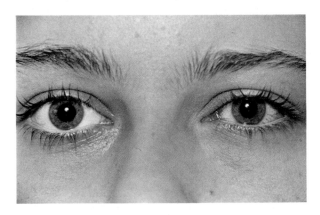

Fig 3-15   Epidemic keratoconjunctivitis. Both eyes of the same patient as in Figure 3-13. Pseudoptosis on the left. Swelling of the semilunar fold and caruncle with minimal conjunctival injection, especially in the fornix on the left. The right eye is still uninvolved.

Fig 3-16   Epidemic keratoconjunctivitis. Same patient as in Figure 3-13. Six days later the inflammation in the left eye is at its peak. There is the beginning of involvement of the right eye.

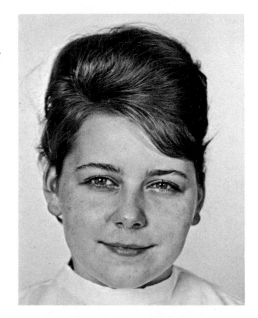

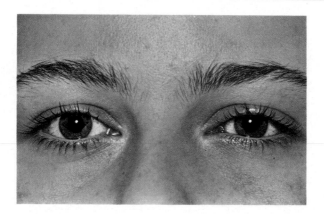

Fig 3-17 Epidemic keratoconjunctivitis. A picture of both eyes shows marked ptosis on the left with considerable swelling of the semilunar fold and caruncle (same patient as in Figure 3-13); beginning redness and swelling on the right.

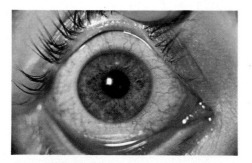

Fig 3-18 Epidemic keratoconjunctivitis. Picture of the right eye (the second eye of the same patient as in Figure 3-17): mild pseudoptosis; minimal swelling and redness of semilunar fold and caruncle. Conjunctival hyperemia especially in the lower fornix.

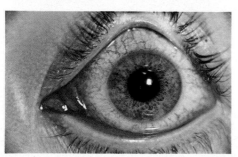

Fig 3-19 Epidemic keratoconjunctivitis. This is the left eye of the same patient as in Figure 3-17. Marked redness and swelling of semilunar fold, caruncle and conjunctiva of the lower fornix (peak of the inflammation). The characteristic bright red inflammatory swelling of the semilunar fold and of the caruncle is remarkable.

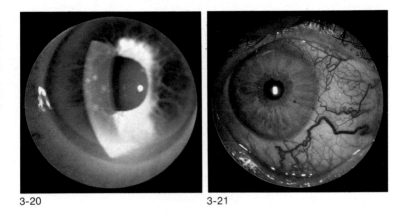

3-20                    3-21

Fig 3-20  Epidemic keratoconjunctivitis. Second stage: epidemic keratitis. When the conjunctivitis has quieted down, there is usually a bilateral involvement of the cornea. However, this happened during the latest epidemics only occasionally. The corneal infiltrates are subepithelial, between epithelium and Bowman's membrane. Initially they are dotlike, later nummular, gray-white, occasionally coalescing. The margins of these infiltrates become motheaten during their spontaneous regression. The infiltrates are usually absorbed completely within a few months (64-year-old man).

Fig 3-21  Episcleral conjunctival venous stasis, after repeated subacute and acute glaucomatous attacks. The pupil is constricted due to the application of miotics. The episcleral vessels are tortuous and hyperemic (46-year-old man).

Fig 3-22  Conjunctival phlyctenule. Gray-red, 2 mm wide nodule, close to the limbus. There is marked local vascular injection with involvement of the adjacent conjunctiva (13-year-old girl).

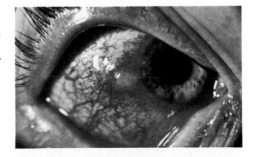

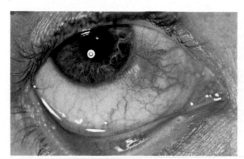

Fig 3-23  Episcleritis. Segmental redness with circumscribed nodular swelling of the episclera. The lesion is tender to touch and lies in the nasal part of the inter-palpebral fissure (43-year-old woman).

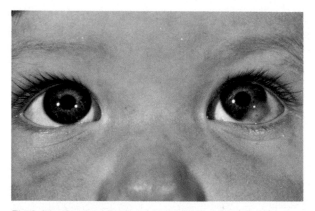

Fig 3-24  Conjunctival epidermoid on the left. Hemispherical, yellow-white tumefaction in the outer lower part of the palpebral fissure. This involves the cornea and contains a few fine hair follicles on the surface. Benign lesion, no tendency for growth (13-month-old girl).

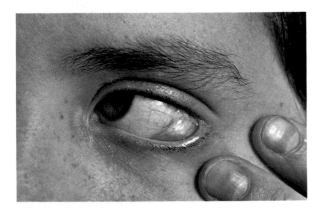

Fig 3-25   Lipodermoid of the conjunctiva. Soft, elastic tumefaction. It lies subconjunctivally in the palpebral fissure, laterally and below, between the external and inferior rectus muscles. The conjunctiva is uninvolved and covers the yellow-red lesion (17-year-old girl).

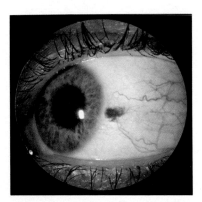

Fig 3-26   Pigmented nevus of the bulbar conjunctiva in the palpebral fissure close to the limbus. The tumor is small, flat, brown and can be moved over the sclera. There are fine cystoid degenerations. The lesion is usually congenital or appears early in life. It is usually benign though it could develop into a melanoma (30-year-old man).

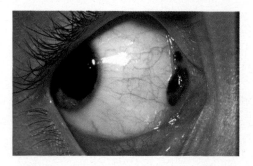

Fig 3-27    Melanoma in the nasal palpebral fissure. This heavily pigmented cystoid tumor lies on the semilunar fold. A satellite tumor can be seen sprouting from the upper edge of the original lesion (12-year-old girl).

# 4. Cornea

The cornea is the light window of the eye. It is an avascular organ and its nutrition requires a complicated mechanism because the limbal vessels supply only the corneal periphery. The epithelium and Bowman's membrane constitute a semipermeable membrane for the tear fluid and similarly the endothelium and Descemet's membrane for the aqueous.

The lack of vascularization explains the vulnerability of the cornea to develop ulcers. In the presence of pathogenic organisms in the conjunctival sac, the slightest damage to the epithelium may lead to an infection of the deep and central corneal stroma. The dense distribution of sensory nerves in the corneal stroma provides an early warning system in the form of considerable pain. This is a type of protective mechanism.

The illustrations show congenital anomalies and degenerative corneal diseases. A frequent example is the senile arcus which in younger patients may point toward an affinity to myocardial infarctions. Other degenerative conditions are the always avascular hereditary types of corneal dystrophies.

Among the traumatic corneal lesions illustrated are the corneal abrasion, bloodstaining of the cornea, the typical corneal foreign body and the painful photoelectric keratitis after exposure to ultraviolet light. Among the infectious corneal diseases are included the epidemic keratoconjunctivitis, the dendritic and disciform keratitis and the corneal ulcer with the descemetocele as an end stage. The rare but chronic Morren's ulcer is probably an organ-specific autoimmune disease.

Other illustrations depict the filiform keratitis as a complication of Sjogren's syndrome, the leukoma of the cornea after recurrent phlyctenular keratitis as well as various stages of keratoconus and its treatment by keratoplasty.

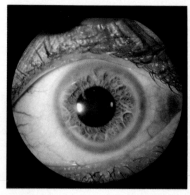

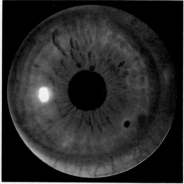

Fig 4-1   Senile arcus. Under the intact epithelium is a narrow gray-white, opaque ring which Is separated from the limbus by a clear zone. The opacity is due to a deposition of lipids. In general, it is an innocuous senile change. Occasionally in younger patients it may point toward a disturbance of the fat metabolism and indicate a certain disposition to myocardial infarctions (31-year-old man).

Fig 4-2   Corneal foreign body with rust ring. For 4 days a paracentral foreign body was present at the 4 o'clock position. Secondary miosis of the pupil with defense reaction: epiphora, photophobia and blepharospasm (28-year-old man).

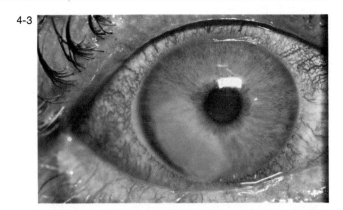

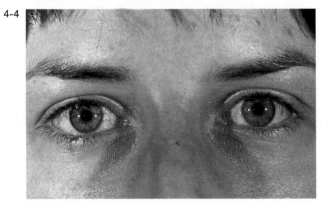

Fig 4-3   Corneal abrasion. Flat denudement of epithelium in the temporal half caused by a lime injury. This area can be stained green with fluorescein instilled into the conjunctival sac. Corneal sensitivity is absent in the injured area and decreased in the adjacent zone. There is pericorneal (ciliary) injection (52-year-old man).

Fig 4-4   Photoelectric keratitis 6 hours after exposure to ultraviolet light. There are fine dotlike epithelial opacities. There is an intensive defense reaction: blepharospasm, photophobia, epiphora and severe pain. The photograph could be taken only after the installation of a local anesthetic (19-year-old woman).

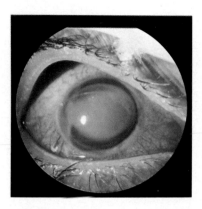

Fig 4-5   Bloodstaining of the cornea after a contusion injury. The surface of the cornea is smooth and there is a clear zone at the limbus. The opacity is disciform, yellow-brown and lies in the stroma. The following factors determine the development of bloodstaining: bleeding into the anterior chamber, filling it at least two-thirds and impedance of the flow of aqueous from the posterior into the anterior chamber or out through the corneoscleral trabecular meshwork (compare Fig 7-4). This leads to a secondary glaucoma. There is traumatic and posttraumatic toxic damage to the endothelium (disturbances of permeability) produced by hemoglobin derivatives (iron) (17-year-old boy).

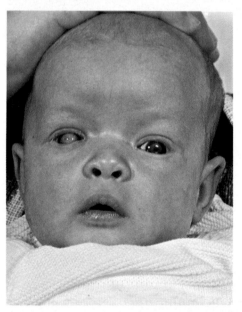

Fig 4-6   Peters anomaly. Congenital malformation transmitted as an autosomal recessive. Central disciform corneal opacities are more pronounced in the right than in the left cornea. The iris is adherent to the cornea in the area where Descemet's membrane is absent (anterior synechia). A secondary glaucoma develops in the course of this disease (6-week-old girl).

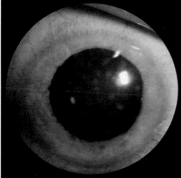 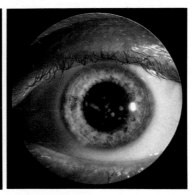

Fig 4-7   Epidemic keratoconjunctivitis, stage 2. Fine, pinlike
subepithelial infiltrates are disseminated over the entire corneal
surface (keratitis punctata super-
ficialis). These infiltrates stain
faintly with fluorescein. They later develop into thin, fluffy
opacities which regress or less
often remain as scars minimally
decreasing visual acuity
(42-year-old woman).

Fig 4-8   Granular corneal dystrophy. Central round, gray
opacities lying in the clear stroma. The corneal periphery is unaffected. Corneal surface and
corneal sensitivity are normal.
Slow progression. Familial oc-
currence (autosomal dominant).
The disease becomes manifest
in the first decade of life. The
cornea remains avascular
(31-year-old man).

Fig 4-9   Granular corneal dystrophy. The entire central cornea
appears cloudy due to numerous
small or large, round, gray-white
opacities. The corneal periphery
is free. No vascularization of the
cornea (22-year-old man).

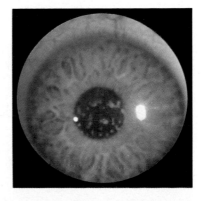

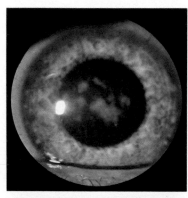

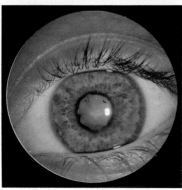

Fig 4-10   Macular corneal dystrophy. This familial disease (autosomal recessive) occurs more rarely than the granular dystrophy. In the pupillary area gray-white opacities are occasionally arranged in a band shape. The opacities are of varying thickness and some of them coalesce to form crescentlike foci. The visual acuity is diminished early, sometimes even in the first decade of life. The opacities increase with time, the corneal surface becomes irregular and there may be loss of corneal sensitivity (25-year-old man).

Fig 4-11   Band keratopathy. Nasally and temporally near the limbus columnar, gray-white, fine opacities extending into the interpalpebral fissure. The opacity consists of hyalin and calcium deposits in Bowman's membrane. This patient had Still's disease with a complicated cataract with adhesions of the iris to the lens (posterior synechiae), see also Figure 5-2 (4-year-old girl).

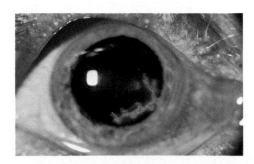

4-13

4-14

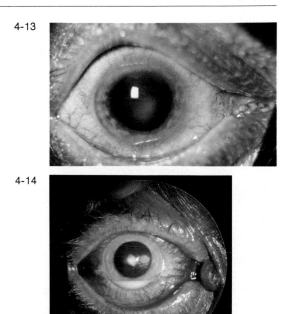

Fig 4-13   Disciform keratitis. This is the deep stromal type of a herpetic corneal infection. There is a central disclike opacity which, because of stromal edema, produces a bulging of the anterior corneal layers. On the posterior corneal surface are folds of Descemet's membrane and fine keratic precipitates. If no epithelial lesions are present, a cautious topical corticosteroid treatment sometimes under the umbrella of a chemotherapeutic agent should be initiated (72-year-old man).

Fig 4-14   Corneal ulcer. Two days earlier a central corneal foreign body was removed. There is now a small, dense, yellow-white leukocytic infiltrate in the central stroma. A progressive margin can be seen at the angle of 12 o'clock. There are cells in the anterior chamber with a 2 mm hypopyon (accumulation of pus in the anterior chamber) (68-year-old man).

◀ Fig 4-12   Dendritic keratitis (herpes simplex keratitis). Somewhat depressed central lesion with branchlike extensions. The lesion stains green with fluorescein. Some of these infections heal spontaneously, most are cured by prompt and intensive treatment with a modern antiviral agent. Occasionally, an abrasion of the affected epithelium may be necessary (42-year-old man).

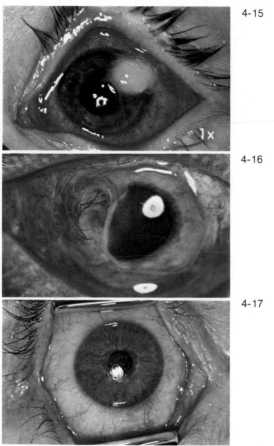

4-15

4-16

4-17

Fig 4-15   Fungal corneal ulcer. There is a dense, paracentral gray-white infiltration. The infection has led to necrosis and the formation of an abscess. There is a feathery border against normal corneal tissue (somewhat obscured by mucous threads). Infection with *C. albicans* after a dendritic keratitis had been treated for a long time with corticosteroids (5-year-old girl).

Fig 4-16   Mooren's ulcer. This geographic ulcer extends from the limbus. It is sharply delineated against the normal corneal tissue by a slightly elevated, centrally undermined gray infiltration line. Painful lesion, irregular progression. The cornea does not perforate. From the limbus a vascularized tissue extends over the irregular ulcerated area. The condition is occasionally bilateral and affects patients in advanced age. It is probably an autoimmune process (73-year-old man).

Fig 4-17   Filiform keratitis in Sjogren's syndrome. The epithelium is rubbed off the basement membrane by blinking. Remnants of the torn off epithelium still hang on the cornea. The denuded areas stain with rose Bengal (74-year-old woman).

Fig 4-18   Keratoconus. The central part of the cornea is thin. The peak of the cone is somewhat flattened and slightly opaque (15-year-old girl).

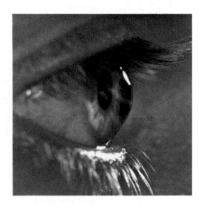

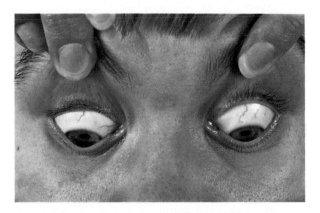

Fig 4-19   Keratoconus. When the patient looks downward the cone-shaped protrusion of the right cornea bulges the lower lid forward (Munsen sign) (20-year-old woman).

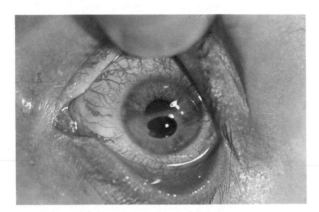

Fig 4-20   Descemetocele. In a patient with acute keratoconus the corneal stroma has melted away and the posterior elastic membrane (Descemet's membrane) is pushed forward by the intraocular pressure. It appears as a black hemisphere protruding over the surface. The central and lower thirds of the stroma are opaque due to edema (28-year-old woman).

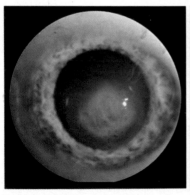

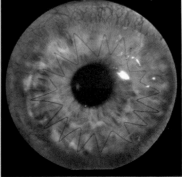

Fig 4-21   Acute keratoconus. Marked protrusion of the thinned corneal stroma. The center shows a dense gray-white opacity due to edema (30-year-old man).

Fig 4-22   Keratoplasty in an eye with acute keratoconus. Continuous suture with a monofilament suture which can be removed after 8-12 months (30-year-old man).

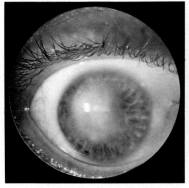

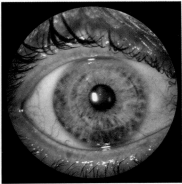

Fig 4-23   Corneal leukoma. Central dense corneal opacity after an attack of phlyctenular keratitis in childhood. Only the peripheral cornea is transparent enough to permit a view of the iris (36-year-old man).

Fig 4-24   Same patient as in Figure 4-23 after a keratoplasty. Clear corneal button (36-year-old man).

Fig 4-25   Band keratopathy. Band-shaped corneal opacity in the palpebral fissure running horizontally from limbus to limbus. The opacity consists of coalescing gray-white dots with dark round holes. Deposit of calcium and hyalin in Bowman's membrane. The epithelium in front of it is slightly opaque. This keratopathy occurred in an older patient in both eyes without any ocular reason (78-year-old woman).

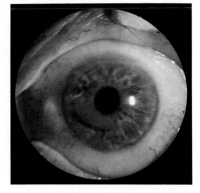

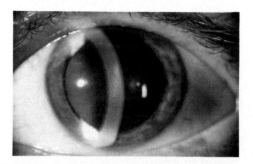

Fig 4-26   Krukenberg pigment spindle. In the central part of the posterior corneal surface is a vertical, spindle-shaped, brown-red accumulation of pigment. This may occur in both eyes and is frequently symmetrical. It is a degenerative phenomenon in older patients and occurs frequently in myopia but rarely in pigmentary glaucoma. Occasionally, it is seen as a genetically determined phenomenon. It can also be seen in connection with cornea guttata (wartlike excrescences of Descemet's membrane) (55-year-old woman).

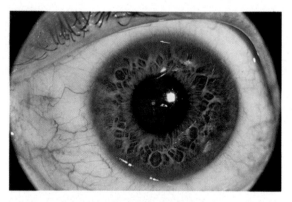

Fig 4-27   Kayser-Fleischer ring in hepatolenticular degeneration (Wilson's disease). A multicolored, 1.7-3 mm wide, olive-green to yellow-red and brown pigment ring lies in the posterior layer of the corneal periphery. The ring is wider in the upper periphery than laterally or below. The fine copper deposits lie in Descemet's membrane. This is a characteristic sign of hepatolenticular degeneration. Penicillamine may improve the disease and lead to a regression of the pigment ring (23-year-old man).

# 5. Iris

The uveal tract is a functional unit but can topographically be divided into three parts: iris, ciliary body and choroid. It supplies nutrients to other parts of the eyeball and can be compared to a vascularized sponge. Most of the uveal blood comes from the posterior ciliary arteries which are branches of the ophthalmic artery. Only a small contribution is provided by the anterior ciliary arteries from the rectus muscles. Because of this vascular peculiarity even a small localized inflammatory process in the choroid may affect large adjacent areas. The uveal tract has an important function and pathologic processes in this organ are always serious. They may jeopardize the transparency of the optical media, the visual acuity and secondarily also the intraocular pressure.

Because the etiology of these inflammations is not known, a logical classification of the clinical conditions cannot be devised. The clinical course varies widely and sharply delineated disease entities are not found. The etiology can be determined in less than 20% of cases. For teaching purposes anomalies and diseases of the iris and ciliary body are discussed together, but those of the choroid will be described later.

Among the congenital anomalies and peculiarities the iris coloboma, anomalies of pigmentation and conspicuous contraction furrows are illustrated. Other photographs show the iris nodules in neurofibromatosis and the pigment proliferation at the pupillary margin after long-standing treatment with miotics. Iris tumors before and after surgical excision are also discussed. Examples of inflammations of the iris include acute iritis, hypopyon iritis in Behcet's disease, fibrinous exudates and synechiae, pigment deposits on the anterior surface of the lens, diabetic rubeosis with secondary glaucoma and posterior synechiae in Still's disease.

The surgical peripheral and segmental iridectomies are discussed as a treatment of angle-closure glaucoma. Finally, shown is an iris suture which closes an iris defect after severing posterior synechiae during a cataract extraction combined with segmental iridectomy.

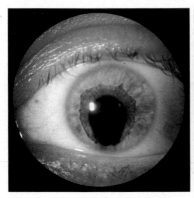

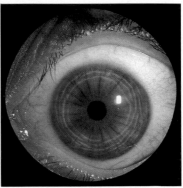

Fig 5-1  Iris coloboma. Congenital segmental defect of the lower nasal iris (28-year-old man).

Fig 5-2  Contraction furrows of the iris. These concentric peripheral rings are especially conspicuous in the hyperopic eye of a child which is shown with maximally constricted pupil (10-year-old boy).

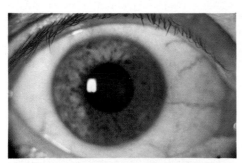

Fig 5-3  Iris of two different colors. Benign, congenital anomaly (37-year-old woman).

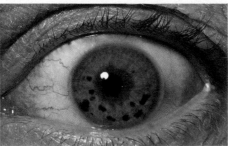

Fig 5-4  Piebald iris. Numerous round, oval or elongated dark-brown pigmented spots in the ciliary part of the iris. Benign anomaly (28-year-old man).

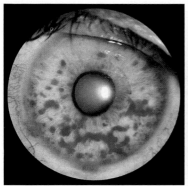

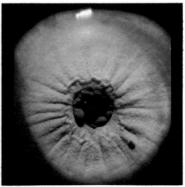

Fig 5-5   Iris in neurofibromatosis (von Reckling-
hausen disease).
Numerous elevated and
yellow nodules in the
iris. The patient also had
numerous café-au-lait
spots on the back
(52-year-old woman).

Fig 5-6   Pigment proliferation at
the pupillary margin. The patient
had used pilocarpine drops for
many years (67-year-old woman).

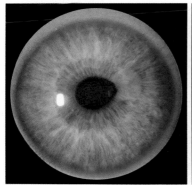

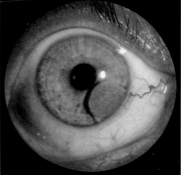

Fig 5-7   Iris tumor. Between 2
and 3 o'clock in the pupillary
part of the iris is a small, yellow-brown, pigmented tumor.
There is a pear-shaped pupillary
distortion. Suspicion of malignant degeneration. The condition
was photographically followed-
up (48-year-old woman).

Fig 5-8   Iris tumor. Nasally below
is a small yellow-brown tumor
with slight vascularization. The
pupil is oval. Gonioscopically the
tumor reaches into the corner of
the chamber (33-year-old woman).

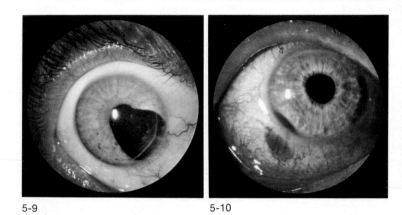

5-9                                              5-10

Fig 5-9   Same eye as in Figure 5-8 after excision of the tumor. Segmental iridectomy. The lens margin and the zonule fibers can be seen in the coloboma. Histologic examination showed leiomyoma.

Fig 5-10   Tumor of the ciliary body (melanoma). The tumor fills the chamber at an angle of 8 o'clock and shines as a black mass through sclera and conjunctiva. The pupil is oval and distorted toward the tumor (48-year-old man).

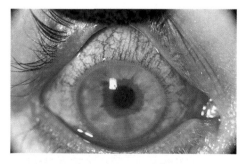

Fig 5-11   Acute iritis on the right. Conjunctival and ciliary injection of the globe; miosis because of irritation of the pupillary sphincter muscle; the iris color is more gray than normal (hyperemia). The aqueous in the anterior chamber is cloudy and contains an exudate (21-year-old man).

Fig 5-12   Hypopyon iritis in Behcet's disease. There is a purulent exudate in the anterior chamber. The pupil is dilated with mydriatics. The disease consists of affections of the mucous membranes (aphthous stomatitis), of the skin (erythema) and of the uveal tract (37-year-old woman).

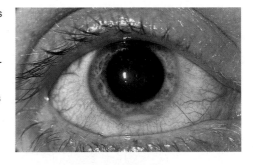

Fig 5-13   Acute fibrinous iritis. Gelatinous exudate in the anterior chamber. The patient had rheumatoid arthritis. There are subconjunctival hemorrhages at 11 and 5 o'clock. These occurred after injection of corticosteroids. The pupil is widely dilated (subconjunctival injection of an atropine-scopolamine-cocaine mixture) (38-year-old man).

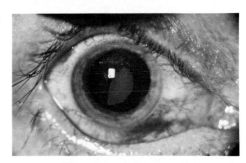

Fig 5-14   Posterior synechiae after acute iritis. The adhesion extends from 4 to 6 o'clock and prevents a wide dilatation of the pupil in that area (22-year-old man).

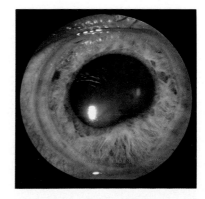

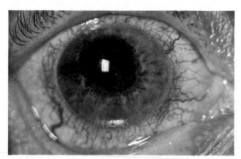

Fig 5-15   Rubeosis of the iris with secondary glaucoma. Diabetic retinopathy. Rusty brown discoloration of the pupillary part of the iris. In this area there are newly formed and dilated blood vessels with a few hemorrhages. At 3, 5, 6, 8 and 10 o'clock a few vessels course from the major circle of the iris to the collarette (55-year-old woman).

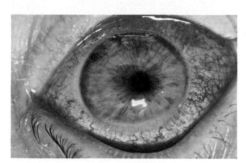

Fig 5-16   Rubeosis iridis. The entire pupillary margin appears red due to a network of newly formed, fine capillaries. Neovascular secondary glaucoma due to diabetes (47-year-old woman).

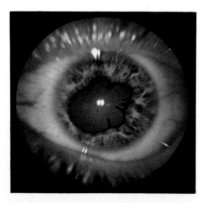

Fig 5-17   Cloverleaf-like pupil. Posterior synechiae after chronic focal iritis. The illumination of the fundus camera produces a red reflection from the fundus (18-year-old man).

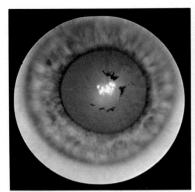

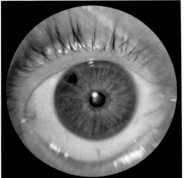

Fig 5-18   Pigment deposits on the anterior lens capsule after broken synechiae. A seclusion of the pupil due to adhesions of the iris pigment epithelium to the lens capsule was broken with maximal mydriasis. The pigment deposits remaining on the lens capsule represent the remnants of the previous adhesion ("footprints" of the iritis). They correspond to the previous location and size of the pupil (67-year-old woman).

Fig 5-19   Peripheral iridectomy after an acute attack of angle closure glaucoma. Triangular peripheral iris coloboma on the temporal side between 1 and 2 o'clock (67-year-old woman).

Fig 5-20   Surgical segmental iridectomy after an attack of acute glaucoma. The resulting coloboma shows at the margins the protruding edges of the sphincter muscle (54-year-old man).

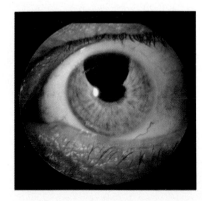

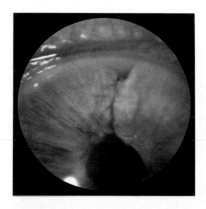

Fig 5-21   Iris suture after the extraction of a complicated cataract. The eye is turned downward. First a peripheral iridectomy was performed and then the posterior synechiae were lysed with a spatula. A radial iridotomy was then placed between the peripheral coloboma and the pupil in order to facilitate the extraction of the lens. After the cataract was extracted the pupillary part of the cut iris was joined by two sutures using monofilament synthetic material (71-year-old woman).

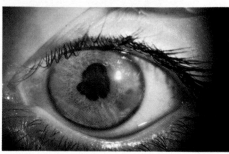

Fig 5-22   Posterior synechiae. Chronic iridocyclitis with band keratopathy in a patient with Still's syndrome. Chronic polyarthritis in childhood. The band keratopathy lies in the palpebral fissure. The complicated cataract occurred after the iridocyclitis. Compare Figure 4-11 (5-year-old girl).

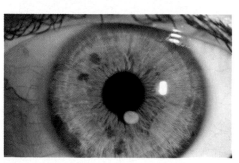

Fig 5-23   Iris cyst. Pinpoint-sized, yellowish cyst at the pupillary margin between 5 and 6 o'clock (26-year-old woman).

# 6. Lens

The lens does not have any vessels or nerves and in contrast to the cornea, the refractive power of the lens varies. However, its elasticity diminishes with age due to the sclerosis of lens fibers in the center (formation of a lens nucleus). This decreases the accommodative power and produces presbyopia though the transparency of the lens may be preserved for a long time.

Congenital lens opacities are often due to a disturbance in the development of the lens. During the early months of pregnancy, the mother may suffer from a viral disease (German measles, poliomyelitis, epidemic hepatitis, mumps) or toxoplasmosis. After the 3rd fetal month the lens capsule has formed and protects the lens fibers. Disturbances in the development or a premature regression of the tunica vasculosa lentis due to intrauterine metabolic disturbances or diseases (uveitis of the fetus) may also lead to congenital lens opacities. Familial, mostly autosomal dominant, congenital cataracts may occur over many generations.

The subsequent illustrations show congenital cataracts (anterior polar cataract, suture cataract, nuclear cataract and zonular cataract) and cataracts due to a German measles infection of the mother during the 1st trimester of pregnancy. The following opacities of a senile lens are illustrated: cortical spokes, nuclear cataract, intumescent cataract and mature cataract (both preoperatively and postoperatively). These are followed by photographs of after-cataracts and intraocular lens implants, which are made of synthetic material put into the pupillary zone of the aphakic eye. Such an eye with an intraocular lens implant is called a "pseudophakos".

Other illustrations show cataracts with neurodermatitis, after lightning, traumatic cataract, the juvenile diabetic cataract, siderosis of the lens and lens luxation in Marfan's and Marchesani syndrome.

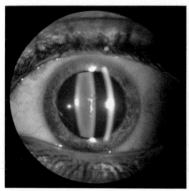

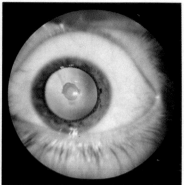

Fig 6-1  Anterior embryonal suture cataract. In slit-lamp examination: white, slightly gray-green, glistening opacity of the anterior Y suture. In the adjacent areas a few dotlike opacities (23-year-old man).

Fig 6-2  Posterior polar cataract. The light of a fundus camera is used for transillumination. A fluffy axial opaque disc can be seen. Fine stripes extend from it toward 11 o'clock. These correspond to branches of the hyaloid artery (arrested regression). The opacity lies behind the posterior zone of disjunction and bulges the posterior lens capsule backward (29-year-old man).

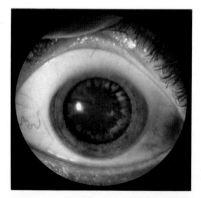

Fig 6-3  Coronary cataract. Club-, disc- and ring-shaped opacities in the periphery of the lens cortex. These form a wreath at the equator and appear frequently blue or green. This is a common type of cataract and occurs in 36% of the normal population. It progresses slowly without usually affecting the visual acuity as the central area of the lens remains clear. It is frequently combined with a cerulean cataract (59-year-old woman).

Fig 6-4 Cerulean cataract. Club-, disc- and ring-shaped opacities arranged like a wreath at the equator. Light blue color. There are also numerous opacities in the central part of the lens causing a slight visual disturbance with increasing age (40-year-old woman).

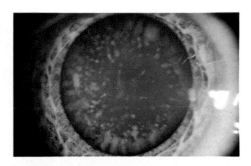

Fig 6-5 Spokelike opacities (senile cortical cataract). Triangular opacities with the apex pointing toward the lens center. The gray-white opacities resemble the spokes of a wheel. Between them water clefts (78-year-old man).

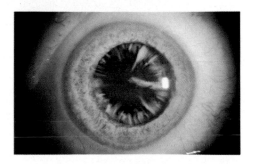

Fig 6-6 Senile nuclear cataract (cataracta brunescence). Dense, diffuse opacification of the brown-red lens nucleus. A few fine stripelike opacities of the cortex (70-year-old woman).

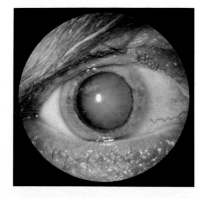

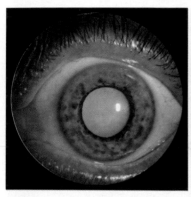 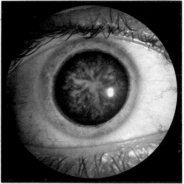

Fig 6-7   Intumescent senile cataract. Due to a rapid retention of water the lens capsule is stretched. The lens cortex is completely opaque with fluffy, milky white material. Water clefts, lamellar separation and vacuoles are only visible in high magnification. Mother-of-pearl shine. The anterior chamber is somewhat shallow. Because of the danger of a secondary glaucoma the pupil is only moderately dilated (59-year-old woman).

Fig 6-8   Diabetic cataract (juvenile diabetes). Subcapsular disciform, feathery spokes and fluffy opacities (snowflake cataract). The periphery of the lens is clear when the pupil is maximally dilated (24-year-old man).

Fig 6-9    Bilateral mature senile cataract. The decreased light stimulation may affect the general health and metabolism of the patient (56-year-old woman).

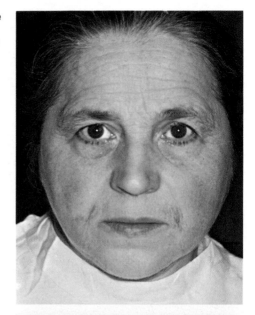

Fig 6-10    Same patient as in Figure 6-9 after bilateral cataract extraction. Considerable improvement of the general well-being.

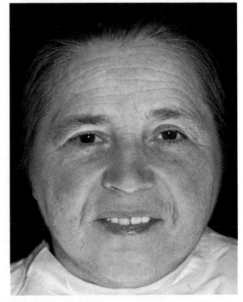

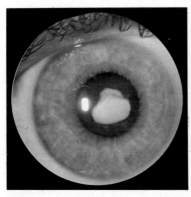

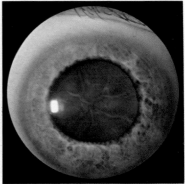

Fig 6-11   Syndermatotic cataract with diffuse neurodermatitis. Shieldlike, chalky-white, axial opacity beneath the anterior capsule in the area of the lens epithelium. A slight indication of radial extensions (11-year-old girl).

Fig 6-12   Electric cataract (due to lightning or electric current). Radially arranged opaque stripes and subcapsular plaques. Water clefts, lamellar dissociation and vacuoles (43-year-old woman).

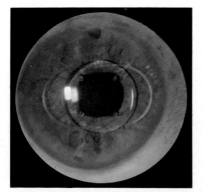

Fig 6-13   Intraocular lens implant (Blinkhorst's iris clip lens). Pseudophakos. The implanted plastic lens lies on the anterior surface of the iris. There are horizontal haptic loops, two lie in front and two in back of the pupil. The connections of these loops to the lens are visible at the pupillary margin as four dots (57-year-old man).

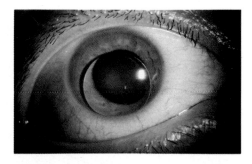

Fig 6-14   Subluxation of the lens in Marchesani syndrome: short stature, spherophakia (spherical lens), congenital subluxation with or without frank dislocation, short fingers. The small spherical lens lies obliquely in the anterior chamber and presses the iris backward. A few zonule fibers remain at 11 o'clock. Secondary glaucoma with luxation of the lens into the anterior chamber (26-year-old man).

Fig 6-15   Subluxation of the lens in Marfan's syndrome: spherophakia, dislocation of the lens, tall stature, elongated fingers. There is an incomplete lens luxation downward. A few taut zonule fibers at the upper equator. Iridodonesis and trembling of the lens with movements of the eye. The anterior chamber is of uneven depth (24-year-old man).

Fig 6-16   Subluxation of the lens in Marfan's syndrome. Same eye as in Figure 6-15. Here the lens is shown in transillumination using the light of a fundus camera. The taut zonule fibers at the upper equator are clearly visible (24-year-old man).

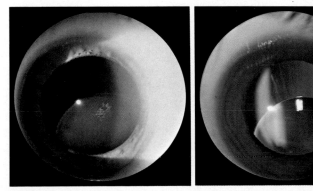

6-15                          6-16

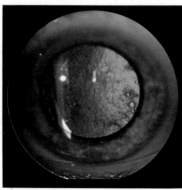

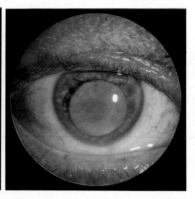

Fig 6-17   After-cataract. In transillumination using the light of a
fundus camera, the Elschnig
pearls and a thin after-cataract
membrane are seen. These followed an extracapsular cataract
extraction (21-year-old woman).

Fig 6-18   Traumatic lens luxation. The opaque lens is luxated
into the anterior chamber. There
is danger of a secondary
glaucoma because the circulation of the aqueous from the
posterior into the anterior
chamber may be blocked
(53-year-old man)

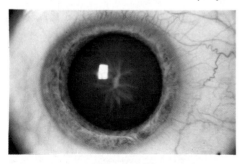

Fig 6-19   Traumatic cataract. Late rosette after contusion. Due to contusion or pressure, the permeability of the lens capsule may be damaged and
the typical subcapsular traumatic late rosette may develop (26-year-old
man).

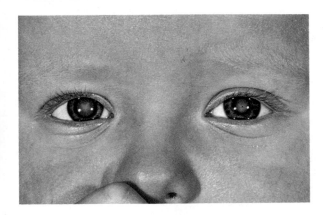

Fig 6-20    Congenital cataract (German measles of the mother). Bilateral, dense, gray-white opacities of the lens cortex. In the 2nd month of her pregnancy the mother had a skin erythema which was interpreted as an "allergy to strawberries." The child has the typical Gregg's triad: cataract, inner ear deafness and congenital heart defect (11-month-old boy).

Fig 6-21    Congenital cataract (German measles of the mother). The cataract was operated on with discission and suction. The child now wears a cataract lens (11-month-old boy).

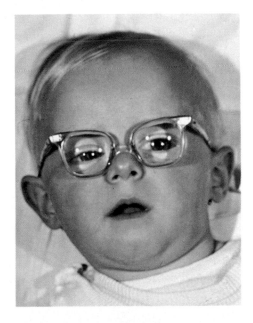

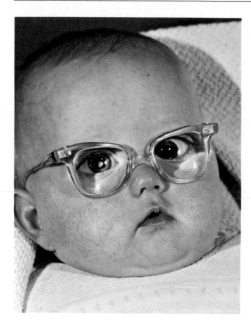

Fig 6-22   Bilateral congenital cataract. The left eye was operated on with discission and suction (6-month-old girl with glasses). The operated eye shows central and steady fixation.

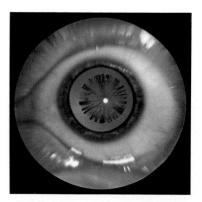

Fig 6-23   Zonular cataract. Saucer-shaped opacities of a specific layer in the lens cortex. The lens periphery is clear. In transillumination using the light of a fundus camera the dark, wishbone-like opaque stripes above a cataractous spherule ("riders") are seen (40-year-old man).

Fig 6-24   Zonular cataract and congenital central pulverulent cataract. Transillumination using the light of a fundus camera. The external saucer-shaped opacity is thin and transparent (zonular cataract). The inner opacity contains a spherical zone with dense dotlike and dustlike opacities (central pulverulent cataract) (10-year-old girl).

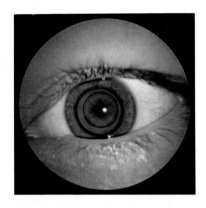

Fig 6-25   Congenital cataract in Down's syndrome (trisomy 21). Lens opacities are frequent. There is a bilateral dense central cataract with clear lens periphery (5-year-old girl).

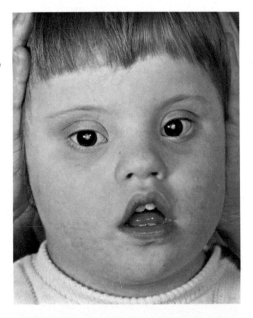

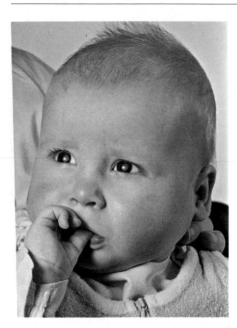

Fig 6-26    Bilateral congenital cataract. The lens cortex is gray-white and completely opaque (6-month-old boy).

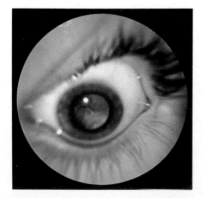

Fig 6-27    Retrolental fibroplasia. This child was born prematurely (the mother was a chain-smoker). Birth weight was 1800 gm. The child was in an incubator for 6 weeks and received supplementary oxygen (up to 30% oxygen). A dense, gray-white vascularized membrane fills the lower pupillary area. A red fundus reflex can be obtained in the upper pupillary area. Vascular loops can be seen in the vitreous (5-year-old boy).

Fig 6-28 Ocular-digital phenomenon in retrolental fibroplasia. The child was born 2 months prematurely. The mother is a chain-smoker. The child was in an incubator for a considerable period of time. (Any prematurely born child exposed to supplementary oxygen for several weeks in an incubator is in danger of developing retrolental fibroplasia.) Both eyes are blind but by pressing on the eyes with the thumbs, the child can apparently produce sensations of light even though the globes are phthisical. Phosphenes. (3½-year-old girl).

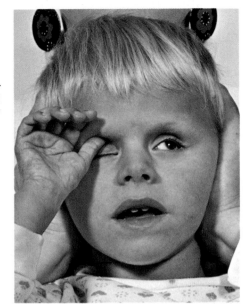

Fig 6-29 Smoking habits of pregnant women. This editorial appeared in the London Times (1974). Potential danger of nicotine damage to the fetus. This is especially critical during the first 3 months of pregnancy, i.e., during the phase of organ formation. The toxins reach the embryo via the circulation in the umbilical cord. The death of more than 10 000 infants could have been avoided if the mothers had stopped smoking during pregnancy. A comparative study on 17 000 children of smoking mothers has shown that not only are maturation and growth retarded, but the scholastic achievement of their children was inferior to those of children of nonsmoking mothers.

## Is it fair to force your baby to smoke cigarettes?

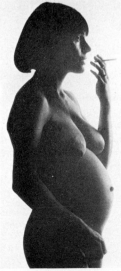

At the present time about 25% of all girls at the age of 10 and 60% of all women at the age of 18 smoke. The offspring of a smoking mother has on average a lower birth weight and a greater vulnerability to infections. Congenital anomalies are more frequent among these children. The incidence of premature birth is 3 times as high among smoking mothers than among nonsmoking mothers.

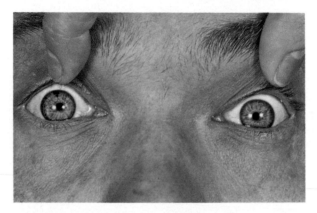

Fig 6-30   Aphakia of the right eye after a traumatic cataract was removed. Correction with a contact lens (23-year-old woman).

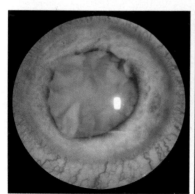

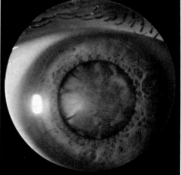

Fig 6-31   Opaque, swollen, fluffy lens material after discission of a cataract. The pupillary area is filled with dense, gray-white lens material which protrudes in the form of large particles into the anterior chamber (15-year-old boy).

Fig 6-32   Siderosis of the lens. Deposition of dotlike and plaquelike rust-brown deposits (iron derivatives) on and beneath the anterior lens capsule. Five months earlier the patient had an unnoticed perforation with a small intraocular iron foreign body which penetrated the lens periphery. Because of retinal damage the electroretinogram is extinguished (18-year-old man).

Fig 6-33  Central pulverulent cataract (bilateral congenital nuclear cataract). Fine, pointlike and dustlike opacities in the embryonal nucleus are seen in optical section. With direct illumination the opacity appears as a homogeneous gray sphere (15-year-old boy).

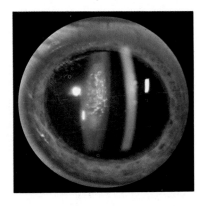

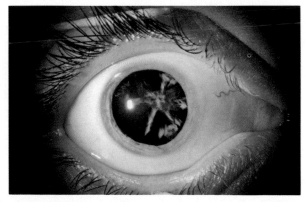

Fig 6-34  Posterior stellate cataract. Both eyes show opacities of the embryonal suture system. The posterior embryonal sutures are surrounded by light yellow opacities. Plaquelike opacities lie close to the suture lines. Some of the opacities are arranged in a feather-like fashion following the course of the lens fibers. This type of cataract is frequently seen in Down's syndrome (16-year-old girl).

# 7. Glaucoma

Glaucoma is actually a group of diseases. Angle-closure glaucoma is an acute form, characterized by a disposition to angle-closure because of an anatomically narrow chamber angle. The hallmark of this type of glaucoma is a painful attack during which the eye is red and hyperemic. In contrast, open-angle glaucoma usually does not produce any symptoms and the anterior segment appears normal. The course is insidious and the disease remains undetected for a long time while the increased intraocular pressure damages the optic nerve. Chronic angle-closure glaucoma lies between the two main categories. In an eye with a moderately wide or narrow chamber angle this variety of glaucoma may begin as a chronic open-angle type and later on develop an acute attack or it may continue as a chronic open-angle glaucoma after medical treatment or surgical intervention following an acute attack.

The subsequent illustrations show in a schematic way the outflow channels of the chamber angle and its gonioscopic picture, the clinical signs of an acute glaucomatous attack, as well as the dilated episcleral vessels which appear after repeated acute glaucomatous attacks or during the late stage of a neovascular secondary glaucoma.

Other pictures illustrate the glaucomatous excavation of the optic nerve head in a myopic or juvenile eye, as well as various stages of the progression of glaucomatous optic atrophy with advancing excavation.

Various surgical procedures for angle-closure glaucoma (peripheral or segmental iridectomy) and for chronic open-angle glaucoma are described. The various filtering operations are shown as, e.g., the classical Elliot trephine or Fronimopoulos's goniotrephine.

Finally, the unilateral or bilateral hydrophthalmus in infants as well as the bilateral hydrophthalmus in mother and child (autosomal recessive trait) are illustrated.

7-1

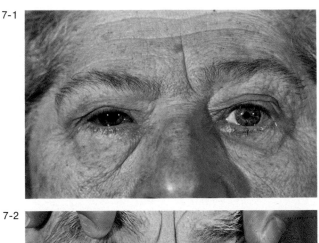

7-2

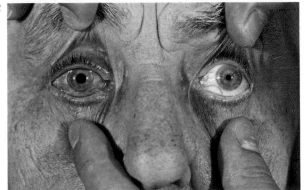

Fig 7-1   Acute attack of angle-closure glaucoma on the right. Pseudop-tosis, congestive hyperemia of the conjunctiva, mild corneal edema; the pupil is oval, barely reacts to light and is wider than the left one. The anterior chamber is shallow. Small cornea with a diameter of 10.8 mm. Intraocular pressure is 60 mmHg. The left eye is white, with a promptly reacting pupil and an intraocular pressure of 19 mmHg (70-year-old woman).

Fig 7-2   Acute attack of angle-closure glaucoma on the right. Swelling of the lids with narrowed palpebral fissure. Congestive conjunctival hyperemia with edema of the corneal epithelium. Anterior chamber shal-low. Pupil in middilatation reacts poorly and despite intensive treatment with miotics is still somewhat oval. Intraocular pressure is 64 mmHg. The left eye is white with open lids and an intraocular pressure of 18 mmHg (75-year-old woman).

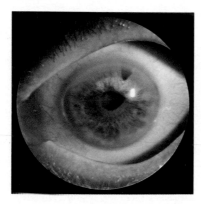

Fig 7-3   Focal iris atrophy after an attack of angle-closure glaucoma. Peripheral coloboma at 1 o'clock. The pupil is oval and the iris stroma shows areas of depigmentation and atrophy. A few stromal strands appear white-gray because of hyalin degeneration (76-year-old woman).

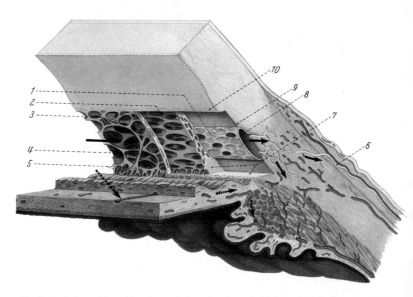

Fig 7-4   Schematic section through the chamber angle (after Thiel). Corneoscleral trabecular meshwork (stepwise dissection) (1-3). The meshwork is a porous structure lying in front of Schlemm's canal and extending between the scleral spur (7) and Schwalbe's line (10). It corresponds to the borderline of the transparent cornea or the beginning of the trabecular meshwork. 4. Uveal trabecular meshwork. 5: Insertion of ciliary muscle. 6: Aqueous vein. 7: Scleral spur. 8: Schlemm's canal. 9: Scleral septum. 10: Schwalbe's ring. Arrows indicate the outflow channels of the aqueous via Schlemm's canal into the aqueous veins. There is also some absorption of aqueous through the surface of the iris and the ciliary body (Hollwich, F.: Augenheilkunde, 9th ed. Stuttgart: Thieme 1979).

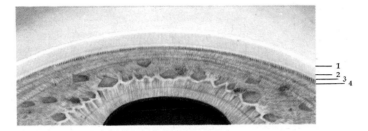

Fig 7-5 Gonioscopic drawing of a normal open chamber angle (after Thiel). 1. Schwalbe's line and above it the adjacent Descemet's membrane. 2: Corneoscleral trabecular meshwork. 3: Scleral spur. 4: Brown ciliary band (Hollwich, F.: *Augenheilkunde*, 9th ed. Stuttgart: Thieme 1979).

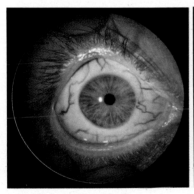

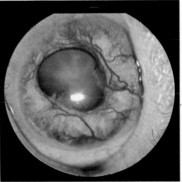

Fig 7-6 Beginning caput medusae in chronic angle-closure glaucoma. After several attacks there is a dilatation of the emissaries with hyperemia of the ciliary vessels and their numerous branches. The cornea is small with a diameter of 10.9 mm. The anterior chamber is shallow with a depth of 2.5 mm (36-year-old woman).

Fig 7-7 Caput medusae. Neovascular secondary glaucoma in a diabetic patient. The pupil is dilated, oval and does not react. The iris is covered with numerous superficial anastomosing dilated vessels which come from the major iris circle (rubeosis iridis). Absolute glaucoma (77-year-old woman).

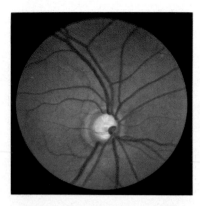

Fig 7-8   Glaucomatous excavation of the optic nerve head in chronic open-angle glaucoma. The excavation reaches the disc margin on the temporal side. There is still a crescent-shaped rim of neural tissue remaining on the nasal side. The cribriform plate is visible and the retinal vessels are pushed nasally. There is marked bending of the retinal vessels at the disc margin. Circumpapillary choroidal atrophy. The visual acuity is still normal, but the visual field shows a marked nerve fiber defect with nasal step (58-year-old man).

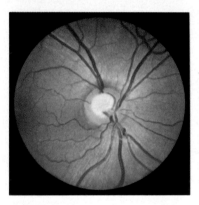

Fig 7-9   Glaucomatous excavation of the optic nerve head. Saucer-shaped excavation with displacement of the retinal vessels nasally. The vessels bend conspicuously at the disc margin. The disc itself is pale and atrophic and surrounded by a peripapillary choroidal atrophy. This atrophy has a yellowish color and may be confused with normal disc tissue. Visual acuity is 0.8. Only a temporal visual field segment including the fixation area remains (53-year-old man).

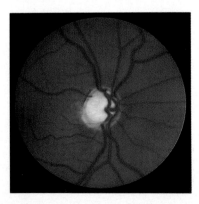

Fig 7-10   Glaucomatous atrophy of the optic nerve head. Saucer-shaped excavation of the atrophic disc with a well-visible cribriform plate. The retinal vessels are displaced nasally and lie at the bottom of the excavation. There is marked bending of the vessels at the disc margin. The peripapillary choroidal atrophy is more marked at 6 o'clock. Visual acuity is only 0.1, eccentrically. Only a temporal island of the visual field remains (55-year-old man).

Fig 7-11  Glaucomatous excavation of the optic nerve in a young
patient. Early stage in a myopic
eye. There is a flat excavation of
the disc toward the temporal
margin in the central and lower
segments of the disc. There is a
slight bending of two vessels
crossing the disc margin temporally. Visual acuity and field are
normal. The intraocular pressure
at 8 A.M. varies between 22 and
26 mmHg (26-year-old woman).

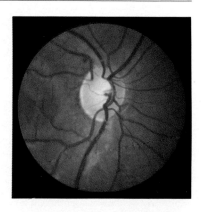

Fig 7-12  Glaucomatous atrophy
of the optic nerve head in high
myopia. The disc is surrounded
by a zone of pigment epithelial
atrophy. There is a flat excavation. The temporal disc margin
is sharply delineated. The retinal
vessels are attenuated and displaced nasally. There is high
axial myopia (-28 D) and chronic
open-angle glaucoma. The intraocular pressure is higher than
22 mmHg only during the morning hours (37-year-old woman).

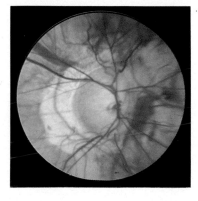

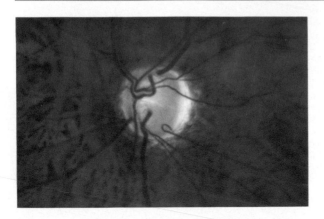

Fig 7-13   Glaucomatous excavation of the optic nerve head. Central, flat excavation with marked bending of the retinal vessels at the disc margin. Total optic atrophy. Absolute glaucoma as the end stage of a chronic open-angle glaucoma. Marked sclerosis of the attenuated retinal and ciliary vessels (63-year-old man).

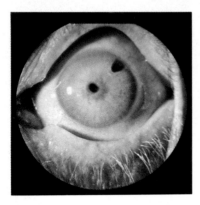

Fig 7-14   Peripheral iridectomy after an acute glaucomatous attack (angle-closure glaucoma). Basal coloboma in the upper temporal periphery. The 12 o'clock meridian is free for an eventual second operation (for a fistulating operation if the glaucoma should become chronic or for a subsequent cataract extraction). There is a small cyst at the pupillary margin. The iris stroma is atrophic especially in the pupillary area. Extremely shallow anterior chamber and small cornea with a diameter of 11 mm (60-year-old woman).

Fig 7-15  Peripheral iridectomy in chronic angle-closure glaucoma. The surgical coloboma is basal and lies temporally. The limbus at 12 o'clock is again saved for a possible subsequent cataract extraction. Because of the advanced age of the patient, a fistulating operation was not indicated. The peripheral iridectomy has taken care of the angle-closure component while the chronic glaucoma can be treated successfully with miotic drops (76-year-old man).

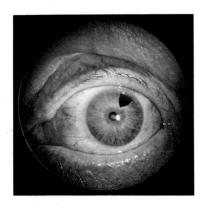

Fig 7-16  Filtering bleb after a classical Elliot trephine. The bleb is flat and the limbal opening can be seen shining through the thin avascular conjunctiva. Intraocular pressure 15 mmHg (58-year-old man).

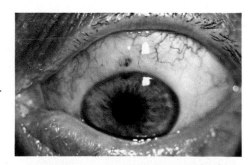

Fig 7-17  Filtering bleb after a classical Elliot trephine 10 years previously. There is a large cystoid avascular bleb overhanging the upper limbus. Intraocular pressure is 13 mmHg (73-year-old woman).

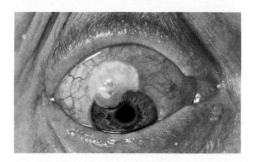

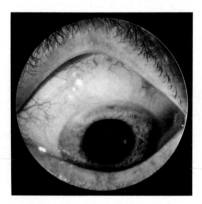

Fig 7-18   Filtering bleb after a goniotrephine (trephine with scleral flap according to Fronimopoulos). Flat, hardly elevated filtering bleb. The trephine opening itself is covered. Three weeks after the operation the pupil is still dilated with mydriatic drops. Intraocular pressure is 15 mmHg (70-year-old woman).

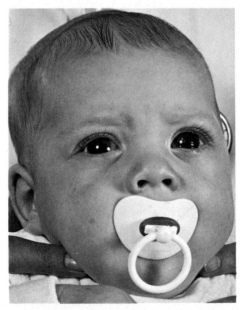

Fig 7-19   Bilateral hydrophthalmus in a boy aged 3 months. Soon after birth the right cornea showed a fine and the left cornea a marked epithelial edema. The right cornea has a diameter of 12 and the left of 13.5 mm. The right intraocular pressure is 26 mmHg and the left is 34 mmHg.

Fig 7-20   Unilateral hydrophthalmus in a girl aged 6 months. The right cornea has a dull surface because of the epithelial edema. The diameter is enlarged to 13 mm and the limbus widened. The pupil is dilated and reacts poorly. The intraocular pressure is 28 mmHg. The left eye is normal with a pressure of 10 mmHg.

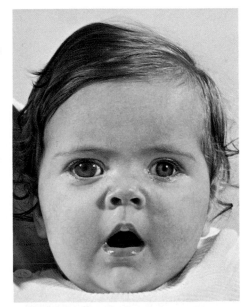

Fig 7-21   Unilateral hydrophthalmus in a boy aged 10 months. The left corneal diameter is enlarged to 14.5 mm. The corneal surface is dull because of an epithelial edema and the limbus is widened. On palpation the left globe feels hard. The right intraocular pressure is 12 mmHg and the left is 40 mmHg.

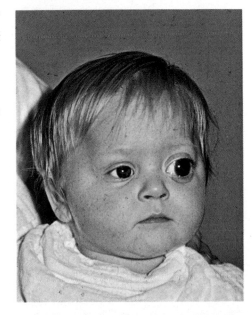

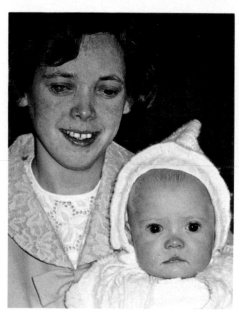

Fig 7-22   Mother and child with bilateral congenital hydrophthalmus. The mother has a blind right eye and light perception only in the left eye (28-year-old woman). The child has right and left corneal diameters of 13.5 mm and 14 mm, respectively. The right and left intraocular pressures are 25 mm and 28 mmHg, respectively (4-month-old girl).

# 8. Choroid

As part of the uveal tract, the choroid is prone to develop metastatic inflammations similar to the iris and ciliary body.

The classical form of inflammation is the recurrent disseminated choroiditis. Among the etiologic factors certain systemic diseases have to be considered, including tuberculosis, rheumatoid arthritis, focal infection, toxoplasmosis (see retina) and others. At present it is thought that most instances of uveitis are due to an allergic reaction. The triggering antigen and the defense mechanism of the body both play an important role in the development of the inflammation.

Inflammations of the choroid are seen more often than degenerative changes of the choroidal vascular system or choroidal tumors.

The illustrations show the fundus in disseminated choroiditis and various stages of a choroidal melanoma.

Fig 8-1  Disseminated choroiditis (recurrence). Small, partly healing, round, occasionally coalescing inflammatory foci are distributed over the entire fundus. There is an accumulation of pigment around some areas of marked pigment epithelial atrophy. Through these the partly occluded choroidal vessels can be seen (41-year-old woman).

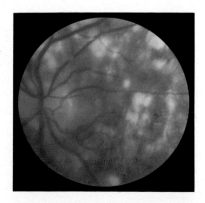

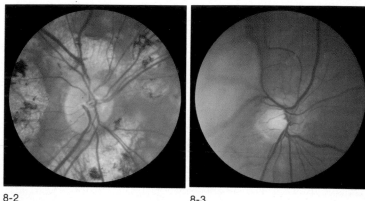

8-2                              8-3

Fig 8-2   Healed disseminated choroiditis. Scarred, sharply delineated inflammatory foci occasionally surrounded by a pigment margin. Areas of pigment hypertrophy are also seen in the scars. In these areas the sclera and choroidal vessels are visible (34-year-old woman).

Fig 8-3   Choroidal melanoma. This malignant tumor extends to the temporal disc margin and rises in a mushroom-shaped fashion into the vitreous. The margins show a deep brown color. In other areas the tumor is surrounded and covered by a secondary retinal detachment (43-year-old woman).

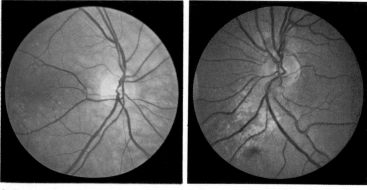

8-4                              8-5

Fig 8-4   Choroidal nevus. (Possible early stage of melanoma). There is a slate gray focus between the disc and macula. It has the size of a disc diameter and contains several drusen in the center. The lesion is only one diameter high, but the irregular surface is suspiciously like the beginning of malignant degeneration (55-year-old woman).

Fig. 8-5   Choroidal melanoma. The tumor lies close to the nasal lower disc margin and has an irregular surface. It is slate gray and shows numerous coalescing light deposits. There is a small marginal hemorrhage. The maximal elevation is 5 D (50-year-old woman).

# 9. Retina: Emboli, Thrombosis

Circulatory disturbances of the retinal arteries or veins produce alarming symptoms. The sudden partial or complete loss of visual function frightens every patient. In addition, most of these patients believe that they are in the best of health and have no premonitory symptoms with the exception of occasional transient obscurations which are frequently ignored. Among older patients local thrombosis is the most frequent cause of circulatory disturbances whereas among young patients true emboli occur, e.g., from an endocarditis.

Only a few decades ago occlusion of the central retinal artery (ischemic infarct) and of the central retinal vein (hemorrhagic retinopathy and venous stasis retinopathy) were conditions which occurred almost exclusively among older patients with cardiovascular hypertension. These days, these pathologic processes occur among young patients and also in women. It used to be assumed that women were protected against these vascular diseases not only by a hormonal defense mechanism but also because they did not smoke. This protection lasted at least until menopause. Today, the combination of contraceptive medication plus nicotine seems to enhance the danger of a circulatory disturbance for women. Many current noxious influences of modern living contribute to the development of these vascular diseases: lack of physical exercise, especially in fresh air, the daily stress of living in a highly sophisticated and complicated environment, abuse of nicotine, a deficient and unbalanced diet, etc.

The sites for such vascular accidents are the physiologic bottlenecks of ocular circulation, e.g., the cribriform plate in the optic nerve head and the arteriovenous (A-V) crossings in the retina.

The following pictures show occlusions of the central retinal artery or vein due to subacute bacterial endocarditis or cardiovascular hypertension. Other figures illustrate arterial branch occlusions in young patients with cardiovascular hypertension and excessive smoking.

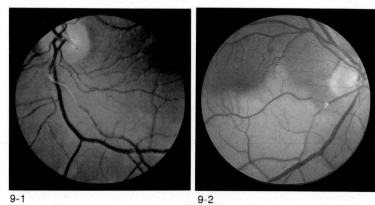

9-1                                                    9-2

Fig 9-1    Branch occlusion of a retinal artery (embolus, late stage). Red-free illumination. Segmental necrosis and extreme attenuation of the inferior temporal artery. The artery is tortuous with focal constrictions and plaquelike deposits on its surface. Septic embolus with bacterial endocarditis (34-year-old woman).

Fig 9-2    Occlusion of an arterial branch with visible embolus at the fork. The retina supplied by the lower branch of the temporal inferior artery is ischemic and shows milky white edema. There is cardiovascular hypertension with a blood pressure of 180/100. The macula is spared (51-year-old man).

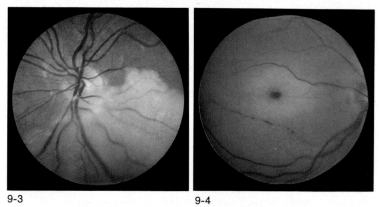

9-3                                                    9-4

Fig. 9-3    Arterial branch occlusion. The retinal area supplied by the inferior temporal artery is ischemic and shows a milky white edema. Cardiovascular hypertension with a blood pressure of 150/95; heavy smoker (24-year-old woman).

Fig 9-4    Occlusion of the central retinal artery. Milky white edema and ischemia of the central part of the retina. Cherry red spot in the macula. Boxcar phenomenon of the circulation in the temporal lower artery which courses obliquely upward toward the macula. Cardiovascular hypertension with a blood pressure of 160/100; heavy smoker (33-year-old man).

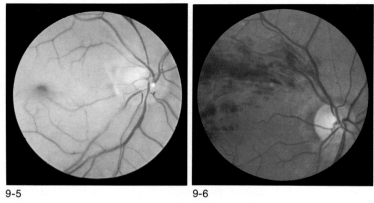

9-5                                    9-6

Fig 9-5  Occlusion of the central retinal artery. The embolus is visible on the disc. Ischemia and milky white diffuse opacification due to edema of the retina. Cherry red spot in the macula (51-year-old woman).

Fig 9-6  Branch vein occlusion. A branch of the superior temporal vein is occluded. There is a wedge-shaped hemorrhage originating from the crossing of this vein with an artery. The retina is edematous and the arteries are attenuated. Blood pressure of 190/120 (52-year-old woman).

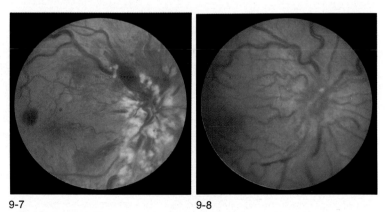

9-7                                    9-8

Fig 9-7  Occlusion of the central retinal vein (late stage, hemorrhagic retinopathy). Dotlike and flame-shaped retinal hemorrhages reaching into the far periphery. The disc is nearly obscured by hard, lipid exudates and cotton-wool patches. Macular edema; cardiovascular hypertension; blood pressure of 160/100; heavy smoker (36-year-old woman).

Fig 9-8  Occlusion of the central retinal vein (hemorrhagic retinopathy). The retina is studded with hemorrhages which reach the far periphery. The veins are dilated. Edema of the disc and the macula. Hypertension with a blood pressure of 140/90 under treatment. Heavy smoker and contraceptive medication. Late complication of a central vein occlusion: neovascular secondary glaucoma (26-year-old woman).

# 10. Retina: Hypertension

This chapter deals with retinal changes which are of special interest to the internist. These fundus pictures are characteristic for various types of cardiovascular hypertension.

There are two classifications of hypertensive retinopathy. In German publications the four stages suggested by R. Thiel are most commonly used. Most American physicians prefer the classification by Keith and Wagener. However, there is no principal difference between these two classifications.

Essential hypertension is one type of high arterial blood pressure. It occurs most frequently among patients who have a characteristic stature. Most of them are short, muscular and often overweight even when they are young. It is a functional hypertension which is for these patients frequently innocuous. The somewhat elevated blood pressure with high amplitudes makes these patients more efficient. It could be compared to a car that has six or eight cylinders. To treat this kind of hypertension by medication and to normalize the blood pressure down to 120/80 might be unnecessary and might affect the lifestyle of these patients in a negative way. However, after the age of 50 these patients should take some precautions, such as trying not to overwork, decreasing the intake of certain food components (salt) and toxins (nicotine) and avoiding excessive activities of any kind.

The following pictures show the various types of hypertensive retinopathy following the four-stage classification of R. Thiel: the benign type in its early and late stages (Thiel I and II), as well as the untreated malignant type in its early and late stages (Thiel III and IV). Thiel was correct in emphasizing that the decisive difference between the benign and malignant types of hypertension is not only the typical vascular change but especially the changes of the optic nerve head. The benign type of hypertension is characterized by a disc which always has sharp margins though it may contain hemorrhages and lipid deposits.

In malignant hypertension there is a mild ischemic early in the course and later a pronounced disc edema. In addition, there are not only lipid exudates, but also cotton-wool deposits with an increasing edema of the peripapillary retina including the posterior fundus pole. A special type of hypertensive retinopathy is the "Kimmelstiel-Wilson" disease in which an intercapillary glomerulosclerosis of the kidneys and diabetes mellitus aggravate the condition.

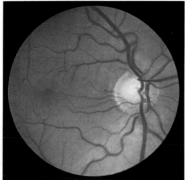 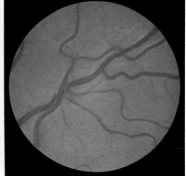

Fig 10-1   Ocular fundus in
hypertension (Thiel I). The disc
is sharply outlined. The arteries
are dilated and of irregular
caliber. Copper wire reflex. Wide
branching of the veins with an
arcuate deviation at their crossing with arteries (Salus sign). Dilated veins. Increased tortuosity
of the perimacular venules. The
entire fundus has a deep red
color. Blood pressure of 150/90
(heavyset, athletic 46-year-old
man).

Fig 10-2   Ocular fundus in
hypertension (Thiel II). The optic
nerve head is normal. Marked
wide branching of the veins
which deviate downward at A-V
crossings (Gunn sign). The
superior temporal artery is conspicuously attenuated. The venules are dilated and tortuous.
Blood pressure of 190/120 (50-
year-old woman).

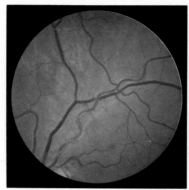 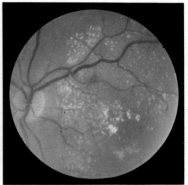

10-3                                    10-4

Fig 10-3   Ocular fundus in hypertension (Thiel II). Sharp disc margins.
Conspicuous tortuosity and variations
in caliber of the superior temporal artery. Copper wire reflexes. Wide
branching of the veins and depression
at A-V crossings (Gunn sign). Increased tortuosity of the perimacular
venules (65-year-old man).

Fig 10-4   Ocular fundus in hypertension. Late stage of arteriosclerosis
(Thiel II). Normal disc. Circinate retinopathy at the posterior pole.
Marked tortuosity of the superior
temporal artery. Strong reflexes from
the arteriolar walls. Conspicuous
Gunn sign: at the A-V crossing the
venule is pushed downward or laterally with banking of the blood distally.
Small hemorrhages near the A-V
crossing. Small and large hard lipid
exudates (69-year-old woman).

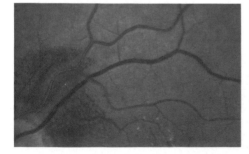

Fig 10-5   Ocular fundus in
hypertension. Late stage
(Thiel II). Wide branching
of the retinal venules with
depression of the vein at the
A-V crossing (Gunn sign).
Flat, superficial retinal
hemorrhage reaching the
margin of the disc. This
bleeding originates at the
crossing of the superior
temporal artery over the
superior temporal vein (pre-
thrombotic stage). Copper
wire reflexes from the arterioles. Small, lipid exudates in radial arrangement
around the fovea (partial
macular star) (76-year-old
man).

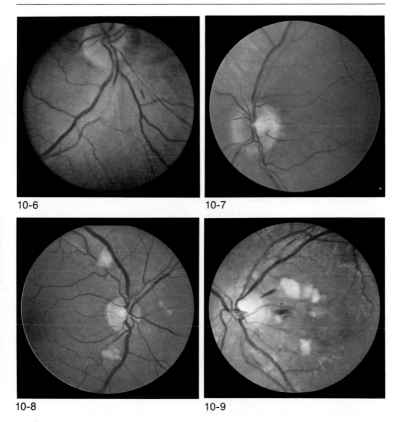

Fig 10-6   Hypertensive retinopathy. Early stage (Thiel III). Delicate peripapillary is-chemic edema. Spastic attenuation of the inferior temporal artery which shows seg-mental hard reflexes. Superficial, flame-shaped hemorrhages. Blood pressure of 160/100 (56-year-old woman).

Fig 10-7   Hypertensive retinopathy. Early stage (Thiel III). Mild disc edema involving also the peripapillary area. Extreme attenuation of the arterioles which are threadlike in some areas. Blood pressure of 170/110 (49-year-old man).

Fig 10-8   Hypertensive retinopathy. Early stage (Thiell III). Mild disc edema best visi-ble with red-free illumination. The arterioles are in some areas markedly attenuated. The relationship of arteriolar to venous diameter is 2:4 (normally 2:3). Between the vascular arcs are two large cotton-wool deposits. Blood pressure of 165/120 (41-year-old man).

Fig 10-9   Hypertensive retinopathy (Thiel III−IV). There is a delicate disc edema on the temporal side involving the adjacent peripapillary area. The arterioles show seg-mental attenuation, especially at the origin of the inferior temporal artery. Ischemic edema of the posterior pole. Two flame-shaped hemorrhages at the temporal disc margin. Cotton-wool deposits at the posterior pole. Chronic glomerulonephritis. Blood pressure of 210/140 (23-year-old man).

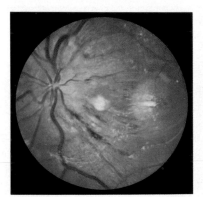

Fig 10-10   Hypertensive retinopathy. Late stage (Thiel IV). Fully developed retinopathy in a child. Disc edema. Ischemic pallor of the posterior pole of the fundus. Threadlike retinal arterioles with silver wire reflexes. Macular star. Large cotton-wool deposit between the disc and the macula. Flame-shaped hemorrhages. Nephrosclerosis. Blood pressure of 250/160 (12-year-old girl).

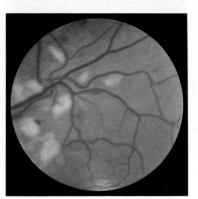

Fig 10-11   Hypertensive retinopathy of pregnancy. The picture shows part of the temporal retina. Mild milky opacification and edema of the ischemic retina. A few dot- and flame-shaped hemorrhages. Numerous cotton-wool deposits among the vessels. Blood pressure of 230/140 (41-year-old woman).

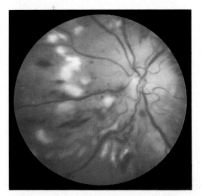

Fig 10-12   Hypertensive retinopathy in Kimmelstiel-Wilson disease (diabetes and glomerulosclerosis) (Thiel IV). Disc edema, retinal edema and attenuation of the arterioles. Cotton-wool deposits and flame-shaped hemorrhages. Blood pressure of 220/110 (30-year-old man).

# 11. Retina: Diabetes

During recent decades there has been an alarming increase in the frequency of diabetes mellitus, which is basically a familial disease. The evaluation of the diabetic retinal microangiopathy has become a most important component of the general evaluation of a diabetic patient from the viewpoint of an internist. This applies especially to the insulin-dependent juvenile diabetics who acquire retinal changes early. These may endanger the visual function. The development of a diabetic retinopathy runs parallel with the metabolic disturbance and the retinal findings are important indicators as to the effectiveness and success of a certain therapy.

Despite intensive multidisciplinary research endeavors and despite the good results of light and laser coagulation, diabetic retinopathy is still one of the most frequent causes of blindness in adults. Another dangerous late complication of diabetes is the rubeosis iridis and the neovascularization in the chamber angle leading to a severe secondary glaucoma (compare Figures 5-15 and 5-16).

*Stage I:* Background diabetic retinopathy. Microaneurysms, pointlike to dotlike hemorrhages. Increased tortuosity and branching of the retinal venules (especially in juvenile diabetes). The veins are hyperemic and show saccular aneurysmatic dilatations.

*Stage II:* Exudative diabetic retinopathy. Flame-shaped hemorrhages and hard exudates (consisting of fibrin, lipid and protein). These appear singly or multiply arranged in a ring- or wreath-shaped pattern (circinate retinopathy). They lie predominantly at the posterior pole. Cotton-wool deposits, i. e., ischemic infarcts of the inner retinal layers with bulblike dilatations of the interrupted axon cylinders in the nerve fiber layer, occur with concurrent cardiovascular hypertension.

*Stage III:* Hemorrhagic proliferative diabetic retinopathy. Recurrent preretinal hemorrhages with bleeding into the vitreous. Caput medusae formation (neovascularization) on the optic nerve head. Vitreous strands.

*Stage IV:* Hypertensive diabetic retinopathy. This occurs in Kimmelstiel-Wilson syndrome. Edema of the optic nerve head and of the retina. Attenuation of the retinal arterioles. Hard exudates and cotton-wool deposits. Malignant hypertension.

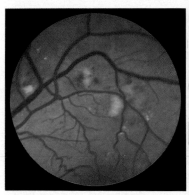 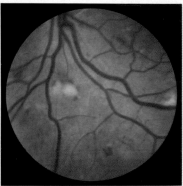

Fig 11-1   Diabetic retinopathy in
a patient with cardiovascular
hypertension. Blood pressure of
160/90. The optic nerve head is
normal. The veins are hyperemic
and partly dilated. Increased tortuosity of the venules. Large cotton-wool deposits with irregular
margins. Dot- and flame-shaped
hemorrhages. Several mic-
roaneurysms resembling small
bleedings. A few round lipid deposits. Stage II (49-year-old man).

Fig 11-2   Diabetic retinopathy in
a patient with cardiovascular
hypertension. Same patient as in
Figure 11-7. Temporal lower
periphery. Marked hyperemia of
the veins which appear deep red.
Flame-shaped and dot hemorrhages. Three large cotton-wool
deposits. Stage II.

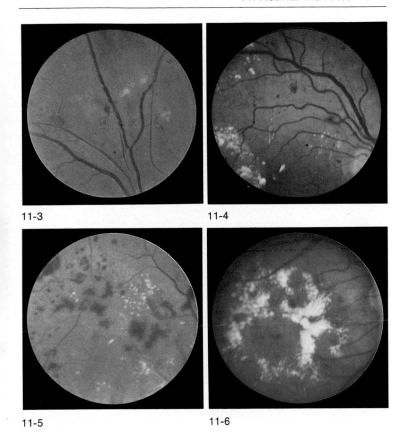

11-3                        11-4

11-5                        11-6

Fig 11-3  Diabetic retinopathy. The optic nerve head is normal. Mi-croaneurysms. Aneurysmatic dilatations of two vein branches. Lipid de-posits and ischemic retinal areas. Stage I (54-year-old woman).

Fig 11-4  Diabetic retinopathy (senile diabetes). The optic nerve head is normal. Increased filling and variations of caliber of the veins. Marked tor-tuosity of the venules. Blot and dot hemorrhages. Lipid deposits. Macular star. Stage II (69-year-old woman).

Fig 11-5  Diabetic retinopathy in juvenile diabetes. The retina at the post-erior pole is edematous, opaque and studded with dot and blot hemor-rhages. There are a few lipid deposits. Stage II (20-year-old man).

Fig 11-6  Diabetic retinopathy (senile diabetes). The optic nerve head is normal. Circinate retinopathy at the posterior pole. A few small micro-aneurysms. Stage II (66-year-old woman).

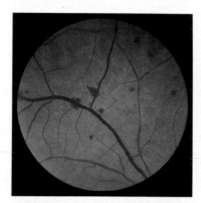

Fig 11-7   Diabetic retinopathy (senile diabetes). Dilated veins with irregular caliber. Thickening of the arteriolar walls. Segmental attenuation of the arterioles. Numerous blot and dot hemorrhages. Stage I (59-year-old man).

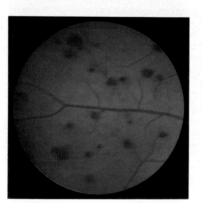

Fig 11-8   Diabetic retinopathy (senile diabetes). Conspicuous variations in the caliber of the large veins. The venules show increased tortuosity. Retina is studded with dot and blot hemorrhages. Stage I (62-year-old man).

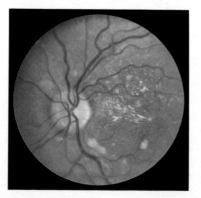

Fig 11-9   Diabetic retinopathy in Kimmelstiel-Wilson syndrome. Intercapillary glomerulosclerosis. Delicate disc edema with marked temporal pallor. The arterioles are in some areas threadlike. Extreme arteriolar tortuosity. A few cotton-wool deposits. Small lipid deposits at the posterior pole. Beginning macular star. Insulin-dependent diabetes for 20 years. Blood pressure of 190/100. Stage IV (42-year-old man).

# 12. Retina: Inflammatory and Degenerative Diseases and Tumors

It must be recalled that numerous diseases of the retina also affect the choroid which is the organ supplying oxygen and nutrients to the outer retinal layers. Many of the disease entities mentioned in this chapter could also be discussed in the chapter on the choroid.

Toxoplasmosis of the retina seems to be an increasingly important entity. The serologic proof of the disease is not always obtainable, but the clinical picture is sufficiently characteristic to make the diagnosis with a reasonable certainty. Senile degenerative diseases of the macula are also increasing due to the increased life span of the population.

The illustrations depict the following conditions: juxtapapillary retinitis (chorioretinitis), juvenile and senile macular degenerations, central serous retinopathy, maculopathy of chloroquine toxicity and angioid streaks with secondary retinal hemorrhages. Finally, various types of retinal periphlebitis are illustrated. Coats' disease and retinal tumors (retinoblastoma, astrocytoma, angiomatosis) are shown and as an example of a typical progressive retinal degeneration retinitis pigmentosa is illustrated.

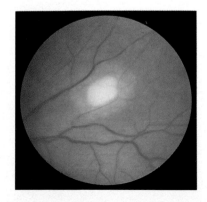

Fig 12-1   Solitary chorioretinitis (clinical diagnosis: toxoplasmosis). Relatively fresh white infiltrate in the temporal upper vascular arc. The lesion is oval, white and about 1 disc diameter in size. It is surrounded by a gray-white, edematous halo. There is only a fine vitreous opacity. Corresponding paracentral scotoma (36-year-old woman).

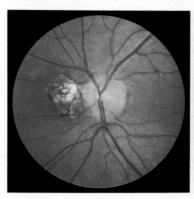

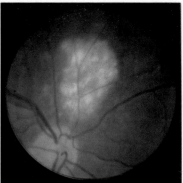

Fig 12-2 Juxtapapillary chorioretinitis (Jensen). At the nasal disc margin is a relatively acute infiltrate (clinical diagnosis: toxoplasmosis). The lesion is round, white and with an irregular, pigmented margin and atrophic areas through which the sclera shines through. The disc is pale and remnants of exudation can be seen in the physiologic excavation. Nerve fiber bundle defect of the visual field. The patient has been treated for 3 weeks with intensive local administration of cortiocosteroids including 12 subconjunctival injections (25-year-old woman).

Figure 12-3 Juxtapapillary chorioretinitis (Jensen. Right eye in redfree illumination. The infiltrate is resolving, oval in shape and reaches the upper disc margin (clinical diagnosis: toxoplasmosis). The infiltrate is white with a few clearing zones. Nerve fiber bundle defect of the visual field (26-year-old man).

Fig 12-4   Atrophic scar in the macula (pseudocoloboma). Congenital toxoplasmosis ▶ in the left eye of the same patient as in Figure 12-3. A large geographic, atrophic scar at the posterior pole is surrounded by a pigmented margin. The scar shows also a choroidal atrophy. This patient shows (with a long temporal interval) both types of toxoplasmosis (congenital and acquired).

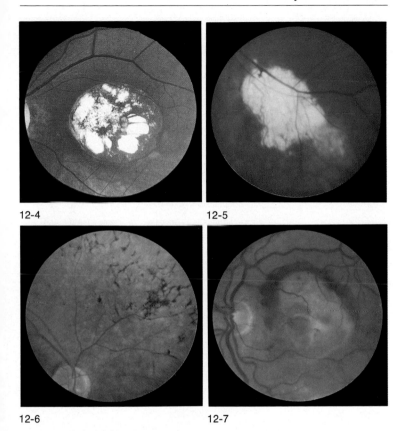

12-4                    12-5

12-6                    12-7

Fig 12-5   Recurrent chorioretinitis. An old, large, white scar (clinical diagnosis: toxo-plasmosis) is seen in the temporal lower area. Next to it is a satellite lesion. This small lesion lies in the temporal lower periphery, is oval, faintly edematous, gray-yellow and regressing (38-year-old woman).

Fig 12-6   Retinitis pigmentosa. A tapetoretinal degeneration. The disc is slightly edematous, waxy yellow, somewhat blurred with a thin pigmentary margin. The retinal arterioles are attenuated and the retinal pigment epithelium is thin. Sclerosed choroidal vessels are visible. Bone corpuscle-like pigmentation in the middle and peripheral retina (42-year-old man).

Fig 12-7   Disciform senile macular degeneration (Kuhnt-Junius). Fully developed picture (wet form). Disc-shaped, irregular thickening of the central retina. White-gray to white-yellow discoloration due to ischemic edema and subretinal fluid. Marginal hemorrhage. Two tortuous macular venules ascend onto the lesion. Marked sclerosis of the retinal and choroidal vessels (75-year-old man).

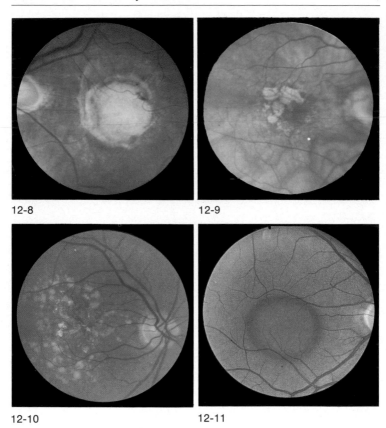

12-8

12-9

12-10

12-11

Fig 12-8   Disciform senile macular degeneration (Kuhnt-Junius). Late stage (macular pseudotumor). Disciform, dense, white scar with atrophic depressed center. At the margin a circular zone of irregular depigmentation. Extreme attenuation of the macular arterioles and venules. The disc shows a senile excavation. Sclerosis of the retinal and choroidal vessels (68-year-old man).

Fig 12-9   Senile macular degeneration (dry form). At the posterior pole areas of isolated, partly coalescing depigmentation. The choroidal vessels are sclerotic and attenuated and can be seen coursing over the bare sclera. Senile peripapillary atrophy with advanced sclerosis of the attenuated retinal and choroidal vessels (79-year-old woman).

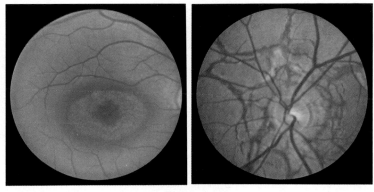

12-12                          12-13

Fig 12-10   Senile macular degeneration (dry form). At the posterior pole are several depigmented areas. Numerous fine, white atrophic foci are present. The choroidal vessels are tortuous and sclerosed. In the surrounding area numerous yellow-brown, round to oval areas of hyperpigmentation over which the attenuated retinal vessels course. The macular vessels are absent. Sclerosis of the retinal and choroidal vessels (70-year-old woman).

Fig 12-11   Central serous retinopathy. Spherical protrusion of the milky translucent posterior retina. The retina opacified by the edema. The macular vessels ascend to this lesion. In the center of the picture a few precipitates are visible on the retina. The patient experienced transitory hyperopia but had good vision with correction. There is a tendency for recurrence. This condition occurs predominantly in men during the 3rd and 4th decades of life (34-year-old man).

Fig 12-12   Maculopathy of chloroquine toxicity (Bull's eye macula). A perifoveal ring of pigment surrounds the posterior pole of the retina. The pigment accumulation consists of fine granules. The center of the lesion appears dark red. The vision was 0.6 on the right and 0.8 on the left. The electroretinogram was normal. The patient had taken chloroquine for 10 years for chronic polyarthritis (35-year-old woman).

Fig 12-13   Bilateral angioid streaks. Brown-red streaks with a light margin extend in a star-like fashion from a circumpapillary ring into the periphery. These streaks are of various widths and somewhat resemble lacquer cracks. The retinal vessels course over them without deviation. The streaks correspond to ruptures of Bruch's membrane. The macula is involved early because of hemorrhages and edema causing considerable loss of vision. The angioid streaks may be accompanied by pseudoxanthoma elasticum (Gronblad-Strandberg syndrome) (33-year-old man).

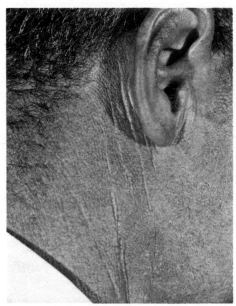

Fig 12-14   Pseudoxanthoma elasticum (Darier). Stripelike degenerations of the skin on the neck in a patient with Gronblad-Strandberg syndrome (angioid streaks). Coarse folds and wrinkles of the skin on the neck and on the forearm. This is a disease of the entire elastic tissue involving skin, mucous membrane and blood vessels. Familial incidence (47-year-old man).

Fig 12-15   Bilateral retinal periphlebitis (Eales disease). Proliferative form at an interval without bleeding, but the hemorrhages recur leading to the formation of strands in the retinal and preretinal tissue. The retinal vessels are pulled to one side and may show bizarre tortuosity. Occasionally they are drawn into the vitreous (19-year-old girl).

Fig 12-16   Retinal periphlebitis. Upper periphery of the other eye of the same patient as in Figure 12-15. Irregularly dilated veins with sheathing. At the A-V crossing and branchings knotty and veil-like, white deposits.

Fig 12-17   Retinal periphlebitis (Eales disease), juvenile recurrent vitreous hemorrhages. Exudative form. Opacification and edema of retina and optic nerve head. Marked tortuosity of the veins with sheathing. Hemorrhages and exudates along and among the retinal vessels. Circinate retinopathy at the posterior pole (25-year-old man).

Fig 12-18   External exudative retinitis (Coats' disease). Frequently seen in young male patients. Usually unilateral. Large areas of white-yellow retinal exudates with a few interspaces of normal red fundus. The entire posterior pole of the fundus is involved. Aneurysmatic retinal vessels and progressive exudative retinal detachment (7-year-old boy).

Fig 12-19   Retinoblastoma. Mushroom-shaped tumor protruding into the vitreous on the temporal side. The tumor is a solid, white, gray mass. Of the patients with retinoblastoma, 25% have bilateral disease. This is a genetically determined tumor with autosomal dominant transmission and incomplete penetrance. The second eye has repeatedly to be examined carefully under anesthesia (1-year-old girl).

Fig 12-20   Tuberous sclerosis (Bourneville disease). Mulberry-like, white, solid retinal tumor. The disease belongs to the phakomatoses (Van der Hoeve). Visual function usually not affected. The tumor originates from the nerve fiber layer of the retina and grows toward the vitreous. One retinal vessel ascends to the peak of the tumor and is 3 D elevated. Incomplete autosomal dominant heredity (34-year-old man).

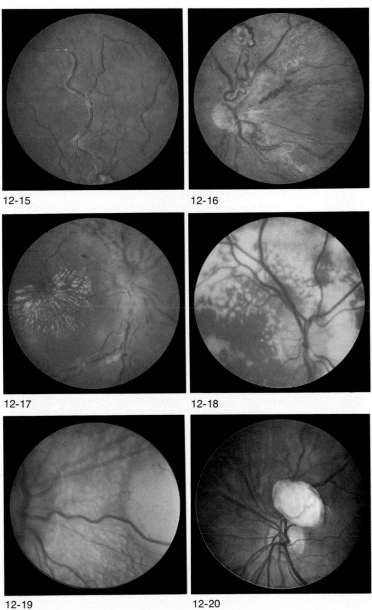

12-15

12-16

12-17

12-18

12-19

12-20

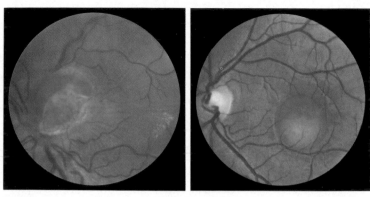

12-21                          12-22

Fig 12-21 Angiomatosis retinae (von Hippel-Lindau). Dark red, spherical tumor which partly overhangs the optic nerve head. The arteries are markedly tortuous and the veins are dilated. Vascular branches lead as afferent and efferent vessels to the angioma. The surrounding retina is edematous, opaque and shows radial folds. On the tumor is a fine transparent membrane. This is a familial phakomatosis. These patients have similar tumors in the cerebellum, pancreas and ovaries (48-year-old man).

Fig 12-22 Vitelliform macular degeneration on the left (Best's infantile hereditary degeneration). An egg yolk-like deposit can be seen in the macular area. The contents seem to be sedimenting downward. Visual acuity is 0.8 and the electroretinogram is normal. The electro-oculogram, on the other hand, is pathologically altered and does not show the usual rise with light adaptation. This disease is transmitted as an autosomal dominant (11-year-old boy).

Fig 12-23 Vitelliform macular degeneration on the left (Best's infantile hereditary degeneration). Four weeks later the contents of the deposit have become liquified and show a horizontal level. Visual acuity 0.6. Same patient as in Figure 12-22.

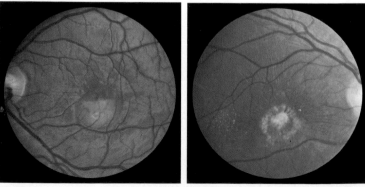

12-23                          12-24

## Juvenile Macular Degeneration

The following Figures are from the **collection of Professor J. François**. The various types of juvenile macular degeneration are classified not according to their time of appearance but according to the site of primary pathologic change.

Best originally described an infantile macular degeneration, which we now know is identical with the vitelliform degeneration. François classifies this as a juvenile macular degeneration although it may be detected at birth. However, most of the patients manifest the first macular changes between the 5th and 15th years of life.

The various types of juvenile macular degeneration affect primarily the sensory retina, the retinal pigment epithelium, Bruch's membrane or the choroid.

All types of juvenile hereditary degenerations of the macula occur symmetrically in both eyes. For an exact diagnosis and differential diagnosis not only is an evaluation of the ophthalmoscopic findings needed, but also a determination of visual function, the electroretinogram, the electro-oculogram, as well as an evaluation of the family tree.

Fig 12-25   Juvenile macular degeneration of Stargardt. Autosomal dominant. The primary lesion is in the sensory epithelium of the retina. The first sign is a disappearance of the foveal reflex. This is followed by a macular lesion consisting of diffuse pigmentation and fine stripes, retinal folds, white dots and a cystoid edema.

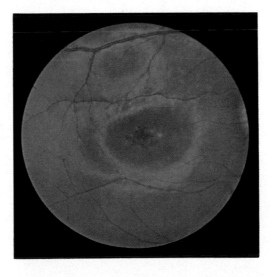

◄ Fig 12-24   Vitelliform macular degeneration on the left (Best's infantile macular degeneration). Late stage: after destruction of the cyst and absorption of its contents, a white starlike scar developed. The lesion is surrounded by hyperpigmentation. There is also atrophy of the retina, the pigment epithelium and the choroid. Vision with correction 0.1. Same patient as in Figure 12-22.

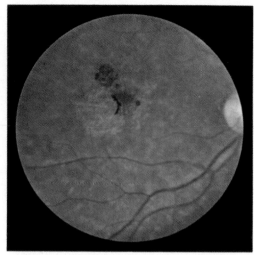

Fig 12-26   Late stage of Stargardt's disease. Central chorioretinal atrophy. The underlying choroidal vessels are visible because of the atrophied pigment epithelium. There is also some pigment proliferation producing the picture of a central tapetoretinal degeneration. In about 50% of the patients there are also paracentral, deep, yellow-brown, fish-mouth-like deposits (fundus flavimaculatus).

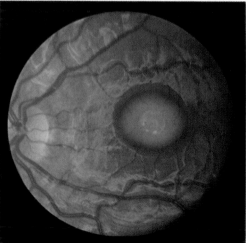

Fig 12-27   Vitelliform macular degeneration (Best's infantile hereditary degeneration). The main pathologic process lies in the pigment epithelium. There is a yellow-red, well-demarcated, homogeneous and avascular disc resembling a fried egg. It lies directly in the macula. This cyst later disintegrates and its contents are "scrambled" (compare Figure 12-23). The end result is a pigmented chorioretinal scar.

Fig 12-28  Butterfly-shaped pigmentary dystrophy of the macula. The primary lesion is in the pigment epithelium. Bilateral symmetrical pigment accumulation in the deeper layers of the central retina and pigment epithelium in the shape of a butterfly. Angioid pseudo-streaks at the posterior pole. Autosomal dominant.

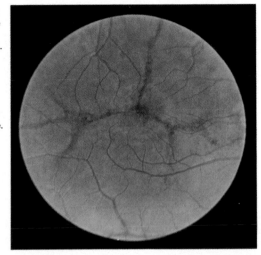

Fig 12-29  Drusen of Bruch's membrane. Hyalin dystrophy of the posterior pole. This may be a degenerative change preceding a dry presenile or senile macular degeneration. Occasionally it is an autosomal dominant hereditary disease (Hutchinson-Tay choroiditis, Holthouse-Batten chorioretinitis, honeycomb dystrophy of Doyne or Malattia Leventinese). Pale yellow, round, deep deposits arranged in a mosaic, occasionally coalescing. Later pigmentation with choroidal and retinal atrophy.

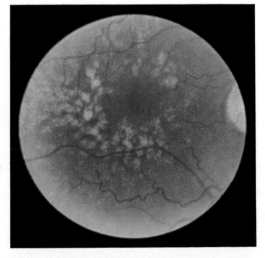

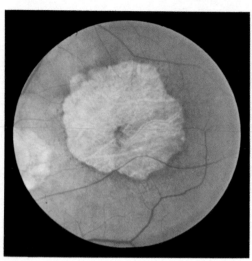

Fig 12-30   Central aerolar choroidal sclerosis. This disease begins between the 20th and 50th years of life with yellowish deposits and irregular pigmentation. Later on there is a progressive destruction of the pigment epithelium with atrophy of the choriocapillaris and the sensory retina. A ring-shaped, yellow-white scar develops. The disease is usually transmitted as an autosomal recessive, rarely as an autosomal dominant.

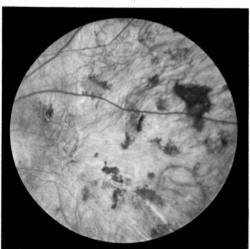

Fig 12-31   Pseudoinflammatory dystrophy of Sorsby. This begins with edema, hemorrhages and exudates at the posterior pole before the 40th year of life. The lesion heals with the formation of a number of pseudoinflammatory scars consisting of white chorioretinal atrophic areas and considerable hyperpigmentation. The choroidal vessels shine through the atrophic scar. There is either regular or irregular autosomal dominant heredity.

# 13. Retina: Retinal Detachment

Only the invention of the ophthalmoscope by Helmholtz (1850) made it possible to observe the light emitted from an eye. This made it possible to examine the ocular fundus and elucidate many diseases of the retina and the optic nerve.

Retinal holes had been observed for many years. However, for 50 years, it remained uncertain whether these holes were the cause or the result of a retinal detachment. Gonin was the first to prove that closing these holes leads to a reattachment. This settled once and for all the prolonged debate.

The examination and evaluation of the ocular fundus has been aided by two important instruments, the binocular indirect ophthalmoscope (Schepens) and contact lenses which allow an exact examination of the vitreous. Syneresis (liquefaction) of the vitreous is frequently seen in older patients. At the same time there may be firm adhesions between the vitreous and the retina. Constant pull and jerking on these adhesions and strands may lead to a retinal tear.

The following Figures illustrate a red reflex of the pupil in high hyperopia, advanced liquefaction of the vitreous, retinal breaks (horseshoe tears and slitlike holes) and retinal vessels coursing over the tears which may lead to vitreous hemorrhages when the retina detaches. The modern treatment of a retinal detachment consists of a scleral buckle (Custodis, Schepens) or encircling band (Schepens, Arruga) combined with closure of the retinal hole by diathermy, cryopexy (Lincoff, Böke), light coagulation (Meyer-Schwickerath) or laser coagulation.

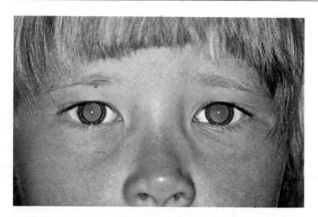

Fig 13-1    Red pupillary reflex. The dilated pupil of a strongly hyperopic eye (7 D) shows a red reflex when illuminated with the light of a fundus camera (6-year-old girl).

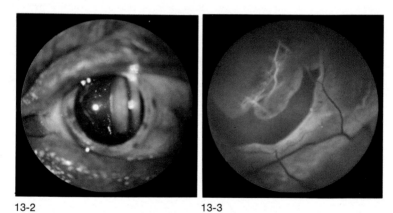

13-2                          13-3

Fig 13-2    Synchysis scintillans. In slit-lamp examination gold-yellow, glistening particles are seen behind the lens. These move with the motions of the eye and then have a tendency to settle in the lower vitreous. These deposits are mostly cholesterol crystals in a liquified vitreous (74-year-old man).

Fig 13-3    Retinal detachment with horseshoe tear. The retina is 12 D elevated. In the right upper part of the picture is a vessel branch coursing freely from the edge of the tear over the deep red to the operculum. The vessel ends in a solid thread. On the operculum a few white, occluded vessels with incomplete holes are visible. Myopia of –6 D (59-year-old woman).

Fig 13-4   Retinal detachment with horseshoe tear. Bullous detachment (15 D) in a myopic eye. The tear is in the upper temporal area at 11 o'clock beneath the insertion of the superior oblique muscle. The tip of the torn off triangle is everted and elevated by vitreous adhesions. To the right a vessel courses over the bright red hole to and through the operculum. Jerky movements and pull on these vessels may lead to vitreous hemorrhages. These hemorrhages may obscure the detachment and make an early diagnosis difficult. This could delay the treatment (use of echography indicated) (50-year-old man).

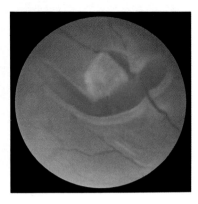

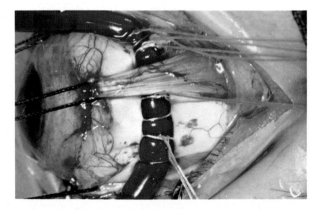

Fig 13-5   Scleral buckle in an eye with retinal detachment. The buckle is beneath the external rectus muscle and tied on both sides. After precise localization the sclera is buckled in such a way that the choroid is pushed toward the detached retinal tear. The preceding cryopexy or diathermy treatment of the tear produces a reactive chorioretinitis leading to scar formation and closure of the hole (63-year-old man).

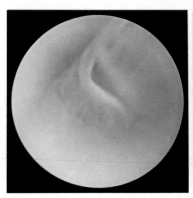 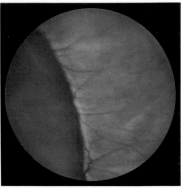

Fig 13-6   Fundus picture 1 week after retinal detachment operation. The slitlike tear lies on the buckle. Cryopexy has produced a grayish white discoloration of the retina. The edges of the tear appear now also gray-white and show a definite tendency to shrink (59-year-old man).

Fig 13-7   Encircling band for an aphakic retinal detachment. A 2 mm wide silastic band is used to encircle and buckle the eyeball. The band lies in the area of the equator and produces a new ora. The small retinal holes are not visible in the photograph. They lie peripheral to the buckle and have again been pushed toward the choroid. The cryo application produces scars which close these holes (28-year-old man).

# 14. Optic Nerve

The optic nerve is a peripheral part of the white brain matter and its anterior ending, the optic nerve head, can be seen with the ophthalmoscope. Nearly 60% of all intracranial tumors produce ophthalmoscopic signs early in their development. These findings are of paramount interest to neurosurgeons. The neurosurgeon Bailey advised every young physician to purchase not only a stethoscope, but also an ophthalmoscope. The fact that the optic nerve is part of the brain explains some of the vulnerability of this structure. The lack of Schwann cells makes regeneration impossible. A disruption of nerve fibers leads not only to a descending, but also to an ascending optic atrophy. Therefore, a diagnosis of "optic atrophy" does not give any clue as to the site of the damage. In order to localize the damage evaluation of other signs is required, e.g., whether the disc margins are blurred or sharply outlined, or other symptoms of defects in the visual field.

The following causes of optic atrophy will be considered: fracture of the bony optic canal, pressure on the optic nerve due to anomalous growth of the bony skull, increased intraocular pressure, syphilis, retinal diseases and vascular and inflammatory diseases of the optic nerve.

The subsequent illustrations demonstrate first the anomaly of myelinated nerve fibers and then various types of optic atrophy: after retrobulbar neuritis in multiple sclerosis, after a fracture of the base of the skull, with chronic open-angle glaucoma, after occlusion of an arterial branch or the central retinal artery, with retinitis pigmentosa and with pathologic myopia (with or without macular changes) as well as with temporal arteritis.

Finally the following conditions are illustrated: drusen of the optic nerve, papillitis, papilledema with intracranial tumor and with marked ocular hypotony and pseudopapilledema in severe hypertensive retinopathy.

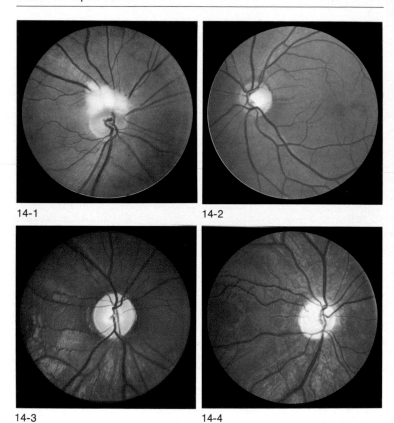

14-1

14-2

14-3

14-4

Fig 14-1   Myelinated nerve fibers. Chalky white, flame-shaped feathery opacities obscure the upper margin of the disc and the adjacent retinal vessels (43-year-old man).

Fig 14-2   Temporal pallor of the optic nerve after retrobulbar neuritis (second recurrence). Multiple sclerosis. Sharply outlined disc with temporal pallor. Flat excavation because of atrophy of the papillomacular bundle and of some capillaries on the optic nerve head (45-year-old woman).

Fig 14-3   Optic atrophy retrobulbar neuritis. Multiple sclerosis. The disc is chalky white, sharply outlined and somewhat depressed beneath the level of the retina. The cribriform plate is well visible. Retinal arterioles are attenuated. The capillaries on the optic nerve head have disappeared (23-year-old man).

Fig 14-4   Total optic atrophy (after fracture of the base of the skull). Chalky white disc with sharp margins. The disc level is somewhat below that of the retina. Marked attenuation of the retinal vessels especially of the vessels in the optic nerve head (8-year-old boy).

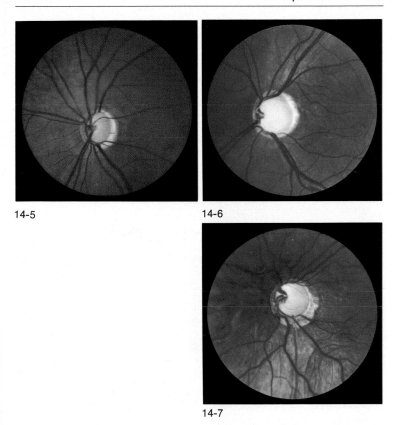

14-5       14-6

14-7

Fig 14-5   Glaucomatous optic atrophy in primary open-angle glaucoma. Only a narrow margin of neural tissue remains on the nasal side. The disc is otherwise atrophic with a deep excavation. The cribriform plate is well visible. The vascular tree is displaced nasally. The retinal vessels show a marked shift at the disc margin. The capillary network of the optic nerve head has disappeared. Peripapillary choroidal atrophy. Vision 5/5 with tubular visual field (61-year-old man).

Fig 14-6   Glaucomatous optic atrophy in chronic open-angle glaucoma. The optic nerve head is chalky white with deep excavation. When the light is focused on the depth of the excavation, the cribriform plate is well visible. The vessels are displaced nasally and show a marked bending over the disc margin. The capillary network of the optic nerve head has disappeared. There is a peripapillary choroidal atrophy. Vision reduced to light perception with a temporal remnant of the field (47-year-old man).

Fig 14-7   Glaucomatous optic atrophy in a patient with bilateral Rieger's anomaly. Deep glaucomatous excavation. Only a small margin of neural tissue remains on the nasal side. There is a peripapillary choroidal atrophy which on the temporal side merges with a myopic conus (17-year-old girl).

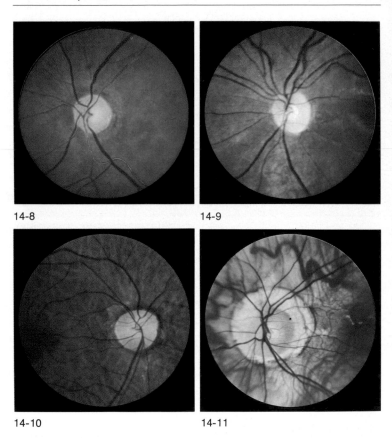

14-8

14-9

14-10

14-11

Fig 14-8   Optic atrophy. Retinal atrophy after occlusion of the central retinal artery. The optic nerve head is pale and atrophic with blurred margins. It is surrounded by a narrow pigment ring. The arteries are thin, sheathed and of varying caliber. The inferior temporal artery shows wide branching, tortuosity and copper wire reflexes. Cardiovascular hypertension with a blood pressure of 180/100 (59-year-old woman).

Fig 14-9   Optic atrophy. Retinal atrophy after arterial branch occlusion. The optic nerve head still has blurred outlines. Only the nasal upper segment is of normal color. The rest of the disc is atrophic and pale. The level of the optic nerve head is depressed below that of the retina. Eight months earlier the patient experienced a sudden occlusion of the inferior temporal retinal artery. This artery and its two branches are recognizable as thin threads. The arteriole coursing toward the posterior pole is occluded (compare Figure 9-3) (24-year-old woman).

Fig 14-10   Optic atrophy. Retinal atrophy in retinitis pigmentosa. The optic nerve head is waxy yellow and because of a slight ischemic edema somewhat opaque. The margins are blurred and surrounded by a pigment ring. The retinal vessels are at-

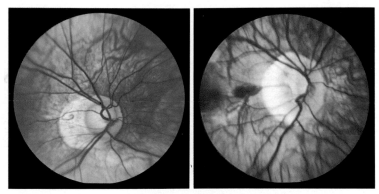

14-12                          14-13

tenuated. There is atrophy of the retinal pigment epithelium so that the sclerosed choroidal vessels become visible. Same patient as in Figure 12-6 (24-year-old man).

Fig 14-11   Optic atrophy. Retinal atrophy in high myopia (–26 D). Due to progressive atrophy of the capillaries, the disc is atrophic and slightly excavated. There is a wide peripapillary choroidal atrophy (myopic conus). The retinal vessels are markedly attenuated and appear stretched. Atrophy of the pigment epithelium with baring of the choroidal vessels. Lacquer cracks in the macula (33-year-old woman).

Fig 14-12   High myopia. Temporal myopic conus. The disc shows a temporal flat excavation. The temporal disc margin is sharp with conspicuous bending of the macular venule at 11 o'clock and slight bending of the arteriole at 8 o'clock. Suspicion of an intermittent increase in intraocular pressure. Retinal vessels are attenuated. Atrophy of the pigment epithelium with visibility of the choroidal vessels (20-year-old woman).

Fig 14-13   Fuchs spot (early stage) in high myopia (–20 D). Circumpapillary conus, wider on the temporal side. A spindle-shaped hemorrhage near the disc at 9 o'clock and a flat hemorrhage in the macula derive from choroidal vessels. Attenuation of the retinal vessels and atrophy of the pigment epithelium with baring of the choroidal vessels (25-year-old man).

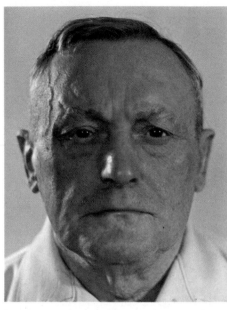

Fig 14-14  Temporal arteritis. The right temporal artery is replaced by a coarse cord which does not pulsate and is tender to touch. Histologic examination indicated giant cell arteritis. Blood pressure of 170/105, sedimentation rate of 94 mm/hr (75-year-old man).

Fig 14-15   Temporal arteritis. Ischemic edema of the pale yellow optic nerve head with blurred margins (same patient as in Figure 14-14). Severe arteriosclerosis with attenuation and variations of caliber. The lower temporal artery is threadlike below the disc. Sudden loss of vision.

Fig 14-16   Bilateral drusen of the disc. The optic nerve head is oval. In the slightly edematous disc tissue are a few refractile, yellow-white spherules (hyaline bodies). Normal vision. Etiology unknown (perhaps interference with axoplasmic flow). Several members of the family had similar ocular findings (13-year-old girl).

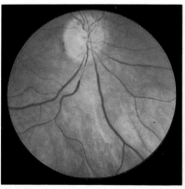
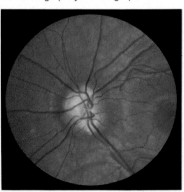

14-15                          14-16

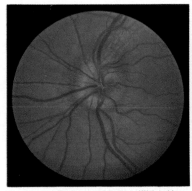
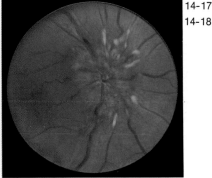

14-17
14-18

Fig 14-17   Optic neuritis (papillitis). Hyperemia and edematous swelling of the optic nerve head which seems somewhat enlarged. The disc margins are blurred. The physiologic excavation is filled by exudate. The optic nerve head is 1.5 D elevated. Vision 0.1 (22-year-old woman).

Fig 14-18   Disc edema with intracranial tumor (tumor of the cerebellopontine angle) Marked edema of the gray-red optic nerve head. The disc is twice as wide as normal. There is hyperemia of the peripapillary capillaries. Fine flame-shaped hemorrhages and cotton-wool deposits at the disc margin. The hyperemic veins deviate when crossing the disc margin. The physiologic excavation has disappeared. The disc is 4 D elevated. Visual acuity is normal, but the blind spot is enlarged (38-year-old man).

Fig 14-19   Disc edema with acute ocular hypotony. The disc is 3 D elevated and enlarged. There is beginning macular edema. The disc edema is due to a postoperative hypotony (intraocular pressure of 6 mm Hg). Spontaneous regression occurred when the intraocular pressure rose to 15 mm Hg (33-year-old man).

Fig 14-20   Disc edema with hypertensive retinopathy. Ischemic edema of the disc (elevation of 2 D). The optic nerve head is twice as wide as normal. The physiologic excavation has disappeared. Capillary hemorrhages in the optic nerve head. The retinal arterioles are threadlike and partly obscured by the edema of the adjacent retina. Dilated veins. A few small lipid deposits and flame-shaped hemorrhages at the blurred disc margins. Chronic glomerulonephritis. Blood pressure of 220/140 (45-year-old man).

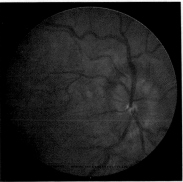
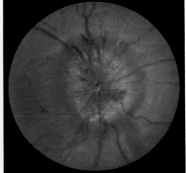

14-19                                14-20

# 15. Orbit

The orbit is a four-sided prism which is open anteriorly. It is filled with the eyeball, optic nerve, extraocular muscles (including the smooth muscles), vessels, nerves and adipose and connective tissue. Any constriction of the bony walls or any increase in the contents of the orbit will push the eyeball forward and widen the palpebral fissure. This will result in an exophthalmos. Enophthalmos occurs when there is diminution of the orbital contents, e.g., with atrophy of the adipose tissue in senescence or when part of the orbital contents prolapse into the atrum after a fracture of the orbital floor. Other causes of exophthalmos are palsy of the smooth Mueller's muscle in Horner's syndrome or flattening of the orbit with premature closure of cranial sutures, e.g., turricephalus.

The paramount sign of orbital disease is the exophthalmos. This may be combined with disturbances of ocular motility usually producing diplopia. An intermittent exophthalmos may be caused by congenital anomalies of the bony orbit (such as in turricephalus, craniofacial dysostosis of Crouzon, mandibulofacial dysostosis of Franceschetti) or circulatory disturbances (orbital varix, Rendu-Osler disease). Damage to the internal carotid artery (fistule in the cavernous sinus) may produce a pulsating exophthalmos. The following conditions may produce unilateral or bilateral exophthalmos: cavernous sinus thrombosis, orbital hemorrhages after trauma, hemophilia, scurvy, vascular diseases (arteriosclerosis), inflammatory diseases of the orbit (orbital cellulitis, subperiosteal abscess, tenonitis, myositis), inflammatory pseudotumor, neoplasms, and other tumors, (e.g., dermoid, hemangioma, fibroma, meningioma, sarcoma, glioma, tumors of the periorbital sinuses, metastatic neoplasms) and orbitopathy of Graves' disease.

The following pictures illustrate the various stages of Graves' orbitopathy which may take a malignant course, as well as the extremely malignant tumor of childhood, the rhabdomyosarcoma.

Fig 15-1 Graves' or-
bitopathy (late stage).
Staring expression, in-
frequent blinking (Stell-
wag). Wide open pal-
pebral fissure so that the
sclera is visible above
the upper limbus (retrac-
tion of upper lid, Dal-
rymple). On looking
downward the upper lid
does not follow (von
Graefe). Bilateral ex-
ophthalmos. Poor con-
vergence (Möbius). Her-
tel exophthalmometer
22/22 with a base of 100.
Reduced sursumduction
bilaterally (69-year-old
man).

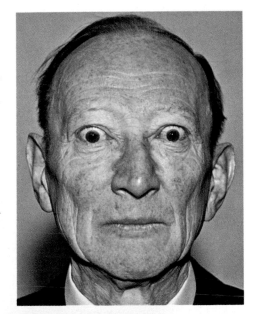

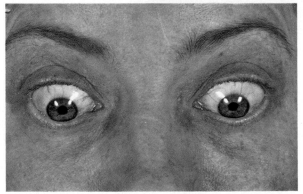

Fig 15-2 Graves' orbitopathy (early stage). Typical von Graefe sign: the
upper lid does not follow the globe on looking downward. Poor convergence when looking downward (Möbius). Increased surface reflection
from the conjunctiva (45-year-old woman).

Fig 15-3   Graves'orbitopathy. Transitional stage to the malignant form. Signs: wide open palpebral fissure with retraction of the upper lid (Dalrymple). Palpebral edema (more on the right than on the left side). Conjunctival injection. Infrequent blinking and therefore inadequate wetting of the cornea. Incomplete lid closure during sleep. Danger of drying out of the cornea. Double elevator palsy on the right (39-year-old man).

Fig 15-4   Orbital rhabdomyosarcoma. Unilateral exophthalmos: marked ► protrusion of the left eyeball forward and downward due to a rapidly growing neoplasm. Decreased ocular motility in all directions with diplopia. Papilledema. Histologic examination showed rhabdomyosarcoma (13-year-old boy).

Fig 15-5   Angiosarcoma of the right orbit. The tumor has broken into the ► temporal fossa. Histologically proved sarcoma. Treatment: exenteration and irradiation (35-year-old woman).

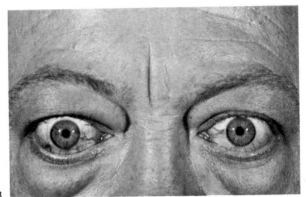

15-13

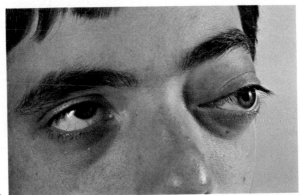

15-14

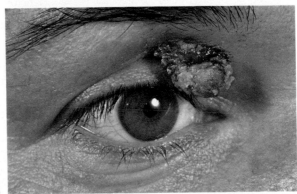

15-15

# 16. Strabismus

Potentially any child can have strabismus. It takes several years before the oculomotor centers in the midbrain and the pons as well as the higher optical centers develop and become stabilized. Binocular vision is firmly established after age five. Before that age, there is a chance that some sensory or motor central disturbance may lead to strabismus. Esotropia usually appears earlier than exotropia. Of all strabismus cases 60% will appear before age two and the other 40% develop before the 6th year of life. The main causes are genetic factors (60%), anomalies of refraction (hypermetropia, anisometropia, acquired poor fusional amplitudes), disturbed coordination or innervation of the extraocular muscles due to hereditary factors, infectious deseases (measles, scarlet fever, pertussis) or birth trauma (hemorrhage into the nuclei of the oculomotor muscles or into the macula).

It is the obligation of every ophthalmologist to prevent during the first 4 years of life any sensory adaptation which may develop subsequent to strabismus in order to avoid double vision. Such adaptation can be either an amblyopia of the deviated eye or an anomalous retinal correspondence (ARC). The prognosis for amblyopia is better than for ARC provided that occlusion therapy or perhaps penalization is used. Under certain circumstances an early operation may be indicated. The straightening of the visual axes of both eyes is a powerful therapeutic measure. The following pictures show preoperative and postoperative examples of esotropia and exotropia. Finally, examples are shown of ocular, compensatory torticollis due to a congenital paresis of the superior oblique. This head tilt develops usually after the 2nd year of life when during the development of binocular vision the patient begins to see double.

Fig 16-1   Esotropia on the left. The strabismus started when the child was aged one. There is now a high strabismic amblyopia with eccentric fixation of the left eye. The deviation measures 40°. The child fights an occlusion of the good right eye. The vision in the left eye is less than 0.1 (2-year-old girl).

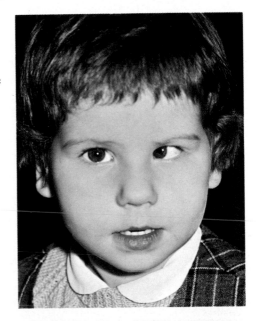

Fig 16-2   Esotropia. The strabismus started when the child was aged one. The good eye is occluded and there is compensatory turning of the head to facilitate a parafoveal fixation of the amblyopic eye. The arms are immobilized (2-year-old girl).

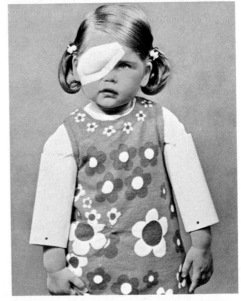

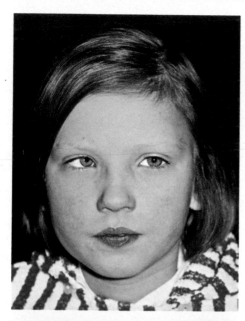

Fig 16-3   Accommodative esotropia. Bilateral hyperopia of + 2 D. Visual acuity 1.0 bilaterally. Without glasses there is a deviation of 28°. Normal retinal correspondence (8-year-old girl).

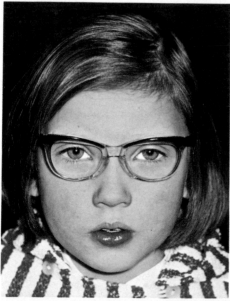

Fig 16-4   Same patient as in Figure 16-3. When the patient wears her glasses the eyes are orthophoric. Normal retinal correspondence with a fusional amplitude from −2° to + 40°.

Fig 16-5 Alternating esotropia. The strabismus started at age 3 months. The child prefers the left eye for fixing. The prism cover test shows an esotropia of 30° and a hyperopia of 6°. The Worth 4 dot and the Bagolini test show alternating suppression. The bilateral visual acuity with correction is 0.5 (5-year-old girl).

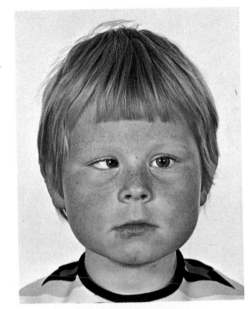

Fig 16.6 Alternating esotropia. Same child as in Figure 16-5. The patient fixates with the right eye. Prism cover test shows 30° esotropia and 5° hyperopia.

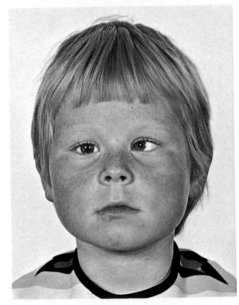

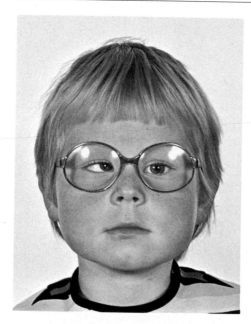

Fig 16-7 Same child with glasses. The patient fixates with the left eye. There is only a small decrease in the angle of deviation to 28°.

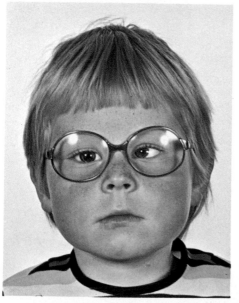

Fig 16-8 Same child with glasses. The child fixates with the right eye and the angle of deviation decreases to 25° and the hyperopia to 3°.

Fig 16-9   Same child after an operation. Six days after surgery there is still an esotropia of 5°, but no hypertropia. Normal retinal correspondence.

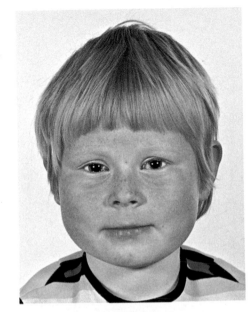

Fig 16-10   Same child postoperatively with glasses. Orthophoria.

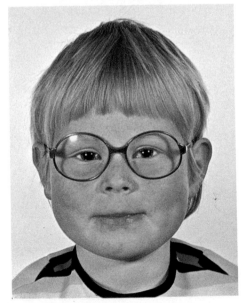

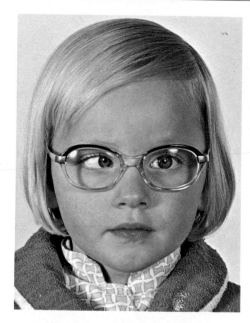

Fig 16-11   Esotropia on the right. The strabismus began at the age of 1½ years. Prism cover test shows esotropia of 30°. Worth 4 dot and Bagolini test show alternating suppression. Visual acuity with correction 0.6 bilaterally (4-year-old girl).

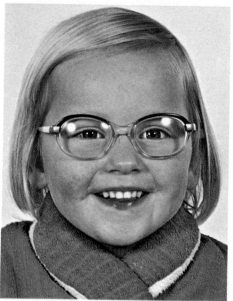

Fig 16-12   Same child as in Figure 16-11 after an operation. Ten days postoperatively there is orthophoria. Normal retinal correspondence.

Fig 16-13   Alternating exotropia. The mother also has exotropia. The strabismus started at age five. The child prefers the left eye for fixation. Prism cover test shows 22.5° of exotropia for distance and 17° for near. Bagolini test shows alternating suppression. Bilateral visual acuity without correction 1.0 (7-year-old girl).

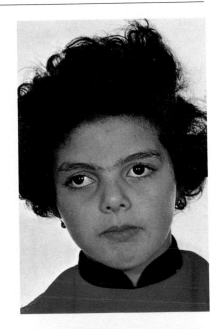

Fig 16-14   Same child as in Figure 16-13. Eight days after an operation with maximal recession of the external rectus muscles (8 mm) and stay sutures. The sutures are tied over the nose and left for 3 days. Eight degrees exotropia for distance and orthophoria for near.

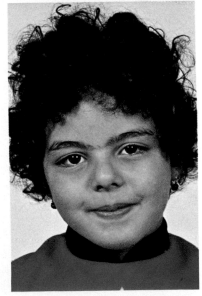

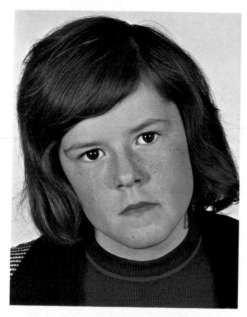

Fig 16-15  Congenital torticollis. Congenital paresis of the left superior oblique muscle. Since the age of two the patient has shown a compensatory tilting of the head. The head is tilted toward the right, i.e., the opposite side of the paretic muscle. The eyes are orthophoric in that position. Normal retinal correspondence with fusion and depth perception (10-year-old girl).

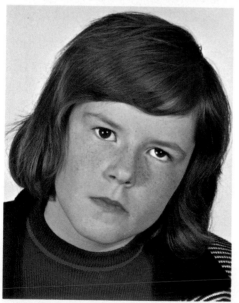

Fig 16-16  Same child as in Figure 16-15. Head tilt test of Bielschowsky. When the head is tilted toward the side of the paretic muscle, there is marked hypertropia with torsion of the left, affected eye. In order to demonstrate the Bielschowsky sign, the patient has to fixate with the right, not the affected eye (10-year-old girl).

# 17. Chemical Burns

Chemical substances, especially alkalines, may injure not only the conjunctiva but also cornea and sclera. They diffuse quickly into the anterior chamber and may produce a secondary glaucoma and lens opacities. They may reach the vitreous and damage choroid and retina. This is especially true for alkali burns which have a poorer prognosis than acid burns, which cause mainly superficial damage.

Chemical burns require immediate treatment. The most important procedure is copious irrigation with water or any other available fluid, e. g., milk, beer or soft drinks. At the same time solid particles should be removed from the injured eye even though this may be quite painful. Any instrument or the corner of a handkerchief can be used. Further treatment should be left to the ophthalmologist who should be called immediately.

The following pictures show the three grades of chemical burns. The first grade is characterized by erythema, but the clinical impression may be misleading. Depending on the intensity of the burn, an anemic edema or the ominous paleness may follow within a few days. It is always important to measure the sensitivity of the cornea, especially in the periphery. Hypesthesia signifies damage to the superficial corneal stroma.

The second grade is characterized by anemic vesicles. This grade usually requires surgery, such as a perilimbal incision into the conjunctiva or a complete peritomy so that the toxic and vasoconstricting exudate can escape.

Necrosis is the hallmark of the third grade, which may be complicated by a secondary glaucoma. A paracentesis of the anterior chamber may be indicated, but the secondary glaucoma responds also to diamox or Timolol. If the pressure can be normalized, a corneal transplant may be performed although the prognosis is not good.

The last illustration shows an eye damaged by an alkali burn. Surgery reestablished the blood circulation.

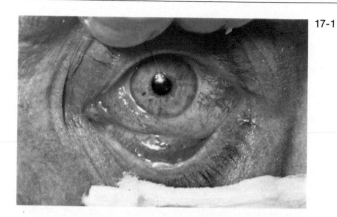

17-1

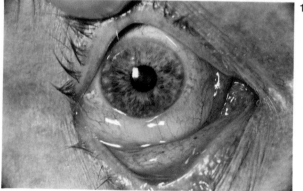

17-2

Fig 17-1    Acute lime burn, 1st degree. Simple erythema and inflammation of the conjunctiva. Mild hypesthesia of the cornea (54-year-old man).

Fig 17-2    Lime burn, 2nd degree. Formation of conjunctival vesicles with exudation. Marked hypesthesia of the lower third of the cornea (66-year-old man).

17-3

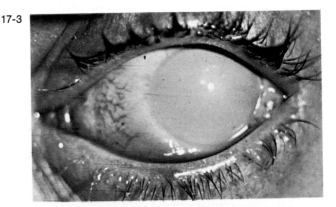

17-4

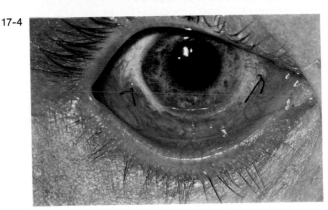

Fig 17-3   Lime burn, 3rd degree. Necrosis and ischemia of the conjunctiva. The cornea shows a dense milky gray opacification (20-year-old man).

Fig 17-4   Surgical intervention for lime burn. Peritomy of the conjunctiva with drainage of the toxic transudate. The subconjunctival fluid has a vasoconstricting effect and its drainage improves the status of the limbal vessels. The incised conjunctiva is anchored to the sclera with two silk sutures (35-year-old man).

# 18. Injuries

Microsurgical techniques have vastly improved the results of treating severe ocular injuries. Monofilament sutures allow a water-tight closure of corneal wounds. Lens material which could contribute to a possible infection and scar tissue formation can be irrigated and aspirated whenever there is a severe injury to the iris, lens and anterior vitreous. If vitreous prolapses into the anterior chamber, a vitrectomy allows removal of the anterior vitreous. . These procedures prevent the incarceration of vitreous or lens into the wound as well as the formation of scars, anterior synechiae and secondary glaucoma.

Injuries at the inner canthus with tears of the lower canaliculus should be closed carefully. Inadequate closure may lead to permanent epiphora as it is usually difficult to correct the situation once a dense scar has developed. The first illustrations demonstrate the clinical picture and the surgical repair of injuries to the lids with tears of the lower canaliculus. The following illustrations depict corneal erosions, hematoma of the lid and subconjunctival hemorrhages after contusions. Blunt injury may lead to a rupture of the sphincter muscle of the iris or to iridodialysis, to hyphema with or without bloodstaining of the cornea and to secondary glaucoma. Hemophthalmos, subluxation or luxation of the lens, Berlins retinal edema, choroidal ruptures, macular holes or disinsertion of the retina are other severe complications of blunt ocular injuries.

Perforating injuries can lead to iris prolapse. Intraocular iron-containing foreign bodies may lead to siderosis of the iris, the lens and the retina. Injuries produced by cuts from a broken or shattered windshield are a special case. In West Germany alone about 1,000 persons annually suffer a blinding injury to one and about 50 to both eyes after such automobile accidents. None of these patients had been secured by a safety belt. These cuts in the frontal or nasal skin as well as into the upper lid and brow are characteristically highly irregular and heal with the formation of a keloid. Cuts of the cornea are of a similar irregular structure. This is due to the fact that the head is usually turned downward after the chin hits the broken edge of the windshield. The cut corneal edges soon become edematous and need a broad-based suture to guarantee water-tight closure.

Another type of injury which has increased in frequency during recent years is the blow-out fracture of the orbit. This fracture is due to a blunt blow to the eye and may occur as a traffic, athletic or recreational injury. The injury causes lid edema and lid hemorrhages. If the lids can be opened, the globe shows decreased motility especially upward and downward. Fracture in the orbital floor may lead to herniation and incarceration of orbital tissues into the antrum. This tissue has to be freed and the inferior rectus muscle (occasionally also the inferior oblique) has to be mobilized and pulled back into the orbit. A defect in the orbital floor may have to be covered by a plate of synthetic material. In complicated cases it may be necessary to open the antrum in a Caldwell-Luc operation.

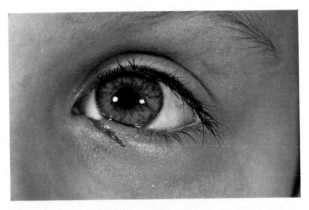

Fig 18-1    Tear of the lower canaliculus by an injury while child was playing. The oblique wound through the lower lid involves the lower canaliculus. Oculoplastic repair includes a resuturing of the canaliculus into which a stent or probe has been introduced ($3^3/_3$ year-old boy).

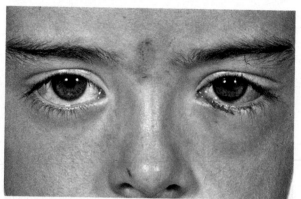

18-2

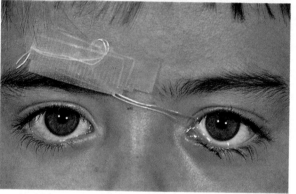

18-3

Fig 18-2   Tear of the lower canaliculus. The patient fell onto the bar of a bicycle. The wound extends close to the palpebral margin from the middle of the lid toward the nasal canthus (7-year-old boy).

Fig 18-3   Same patient as in Figure 18-2. Closure of the wound. The lower canaliculus has been resutured over a probe. The probe has been introduced into the upper punctum and exits through the lower punctum. The stent remains in the canaliculi for 6 weeks. The suture is gently moved every day.

18-4

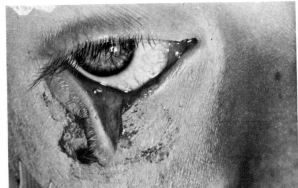

18-5

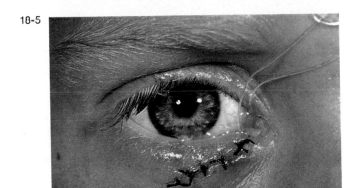

Fig 18-4  Tear of the lower lid with a wire. The wire was stuck into the lid and when it was removed forcibly the inner canthus tore. The torn margin of the lower lid is everted. The punctum is visible in the torn part of the lid (8-year-old boy).

Fig 18-5  Same patient as in Figure 18-4 on the 1st postoperative day. The lid wound was closed in layers. The lower canaliculus was closed over a probe. A stent remains in the canaliculi and the suture exiting from the upper and lower punctum is fastened to the front. This suture is gently moved every day for 6 weeks.

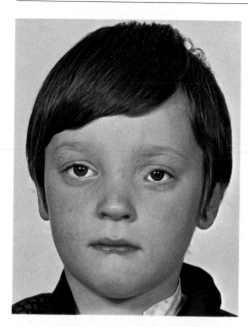

Fig 18-6    Dog bite injury to the lid. The lid wound was closed with interrupted sutures. The torn left lower canaliculus with a subsequent epiphora (8-year-old boy).

Fig 18-7    Corneal erosion. The central part of the cornea has been denuded from its epithelium..The catoptric image produced from this area (window cross) is dull and lacks its normal high reflectivity. The area stains intensively with fluorescein. The bared corneal nerves cause severe pain. There is pericorneal and ciliary injection (61-year-old woman). ►

Fig 18-8    Hematoma into the lid and subconjunctivally after contusion of the globe. The lower and temporal bulbar conjunctiva are elevated by blood. The pupil is in mid-dilatation and reacts slowly because of traumatic damage to the sphincter muscle of the iris. The fundus shows Berlin's edema (24-year-old man). ►

Fig 18-9    Tear of the sphincter at 6 o'clock after contusion of the globe. ►
The sphincter muscle of the pupil has been torn. This may occur when, during impact, the pupil is dilated and the sphincter relaxed and thin. On the other hand, iridodialysis will result when, during impact, the pupil is constricted and the iris therefore taut and thin (36-year-old woman).

18-7

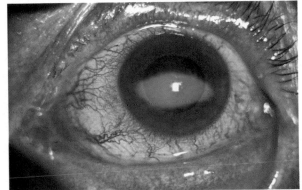

18-8

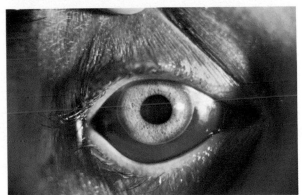

18-9

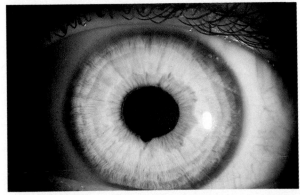

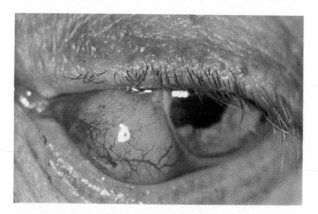

Fig 18-10   Luxation of the lens under the conjunctiva. The lens has been luxated nasally and lies with prolapsed vitreous beneath the conjunctiva. It bulges like a bleb into the palpebral fissure. Indirect scleral rupture when the eye was hit by a log of wood (68-year-old man).

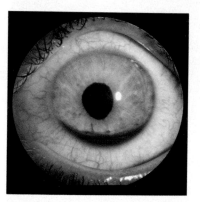

Fig 18-11   Hyphema. Traumatic mydriasis after the eye was hit with a snowball. The hemorrhage into the anterior chamber has settled with a horizontal level into the lower angle (11-year-old boy).

Fig 18-14   Hemophthalmus after contusion injury. Severe subconjunctival ▶ hemorrhage. The hyphema fills the anterior chamber. Blood beginning to stain the cornea (68-year-old woman).

18-12

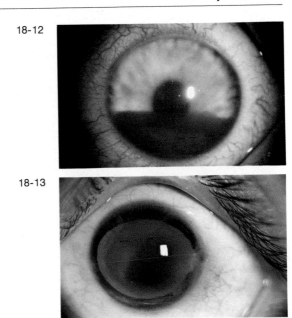

18-13

Fig 18-12   Hyphema after contusion of the globe (the eye was hit by an arrow). The blood in the anterior chamber reaches the center of the pupil. There is corneal edema because of a secondary glaucoma. Due to the tear in the sphincter the pupil is oval and reacts slowly. The blood in the iris produces a secondary heterochromia. The bulbar conjunctiva shows congestive hyperemia and some edema (14-year-old boy).

Fig 18-13   Bloodstaining of the cornea after contusion injury (the eye was hit by an arrow). Six months earlier the anterior chamber had been filled with blood and the hyphema recurred. The corneal endothelium has been damaged by the trauma and by posttraumatic complications (increased intraocular pressure, decreased nutrition of the cells). Hemoglobin and its derivative are pressed into the corneal stroma. Advanced atrophy of the iris (7-year-old boy).

18-14

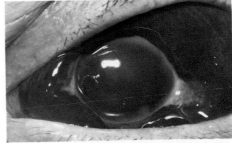

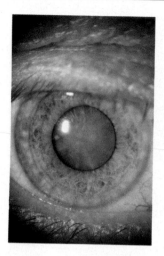

Fig 18-15  Siderosis of the lens. The lens is opaque and slightly swollen (complicated cataract). Pinpoint and flat rusty brown precipitates on and beneath the capsule. The perforating injury occurred 3 months previously with a small iron foreign body. At that time an erroneous diagnosis of traumatic conjunctivitis had been made and no X-ray had been taken although the history had revealed that the patient had hammered on iron. The electroretinogram is now extinguished (45-year-old man).

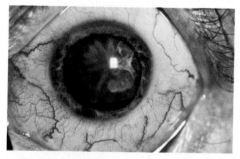

Fig 18-16  Subluxation of the lens after contusion of the globe. Circumscribed, gray-white opacification of the lens capsule. Irreversible mydriasis and irregular shape of the pupil. Iris atrophy (53-year-old man).

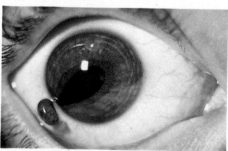

Fig 18-17  Iris prolapse after perforating injury. The pupil is pearshaped and points toward the scleral injury. The iris is incarcerated. The accident occurred 2 hours earlier and the iris tissue has not yet changed its color (11-year-old boy).

Fig 18-18   Iridodialysis after contusion of the globe. The iris is torn at its root between 5 and 6 o'clock. The pupil is oval (19-year-old man).

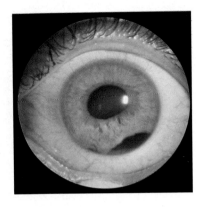

Fig 18-19   Traumatic iridodialysis. The temporal iris is torn at its root from 7 o'clock over 9 o'clock to 1 o'clock. The pupil is displaced nasally and slitlike. Marked photophobia in bright light (35-year-old man).

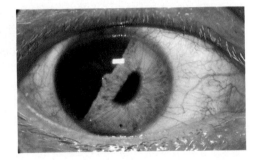

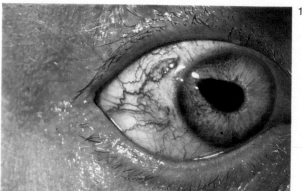

18-20

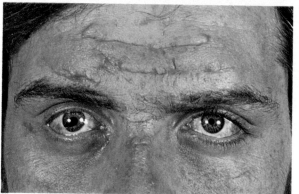

18-21

Fig 18-20   Same patient as in Figure 18-19. The root of the iris has been anchored to the chamber angle by two sutures on the temporal side. Five days postoperatively. The photophobia has disappeared (35-year-old man).

Fig 18-21   Windshield injury. Typical keloid scars cross the root of the nose, the upper lid, the brow and the front. Perforating injury on the right (19-year-old boy).

18-22

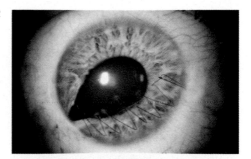

18-23

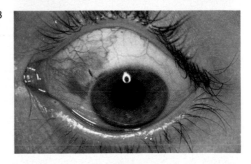

Fig 18-22   Right eye of the same patient as shown in Figure 18-21. Perforating corneal wound closed with a running nontraumatic monofilament suture. The suture is tied at 8 o'clock in the episclera. Pear-shaped surgical iris coloboma at 8 o'clock after the prolapsed discolored iris had been excised (3 days after the injury).

Fig 18-23   Perforating injury with a sharp piece of metal. Small radial, slit-like limbal perforation at 11 o'clock. The scleral wound has sharp edges. The anterior chamber and pupil are normal. The X-ray shows intraocular metallic foreign body (14-year-old boy).

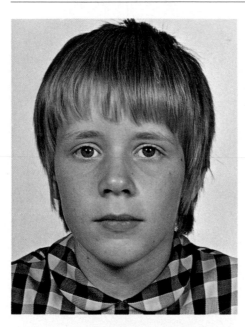

Fig 18-24    Blow-out fracture of the left orbit. Five days earlier the patient had been unintentionally hit by a heel during gymnastics. When the patient looks straight ahead there is no diplopia (11-year-old girl).

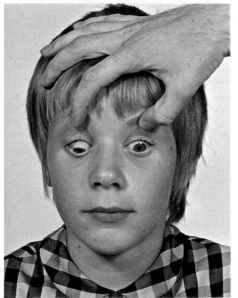

Fig 18-25    Same patient as in Figure 18-24. When looking downward the left eye shows restricted motion. Diplopia.

Fig 18-26    Same patient. When looking upward the left eye also shows a restricted motion. Diplopia.

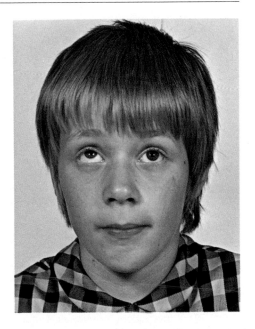

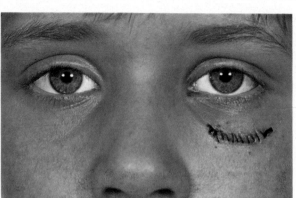

18-27

Fig 18-27    Same patient. Eight days postoperatively. The incarcerated inferior rectus muscle was mobilized from the fracture in the orbital floor. The bony defect was covered with a sheet of plastic material which was anchored to the periosteum. The periorbital tissue was closed with catgut and the skin with a continuous silk suture.

Fig 18-28    Same patient. Plotting of ocular motility on a diplopia screen, ► before the operation.

Fig 18-29    Same patient. Plotting of ocular motility on a diplopia screen. ► Six weeks after the operation.

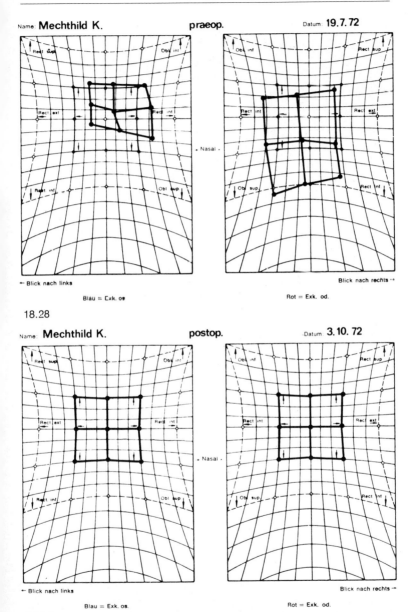

Name: **Mechthild K.** praeop. Datum: **19.7.72**

← Blick nach links

Blick nach rechts →

Blau = Exk. os

Rot = Exk. od.

18.28

Name: **Mechthild K.** postop. Datum: **3.10.72**

← Blick nach links

Blick nach rechts →

Blau = Exk. os.

Rot = Exk. od.

18.29

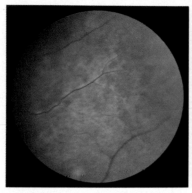 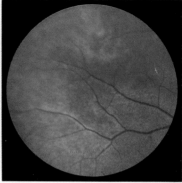

Fig 18-30   Berlin's edema on the left. One day before the eye had been hit by a thrown apple. White-gray, ischemic retinal area in the temporal upper periphery. Perivascular sheathing of the attenuated artery which courses from the center of the picture upward and outward. The peripheral branches are filled with blood, while two branches coursing temporally and down are still nearly empty (12-year-old boy).

Fig 18-31   Berlin's edema. White-gray, ischemic retina in the temporal periphery. Only a small margin at the nasal upper edge of the picture is spared and appears normal. The choroidal vessels are barely visible beneath the retinal edema on the temporal side. The retinal artery which branches in the temporal lower periphery still shows perivascular sheathing. Contusion injury of the globe when hit by a ball (15-year-old girl).

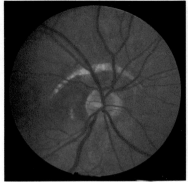 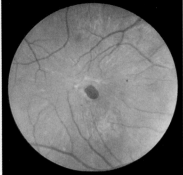

Fig 18-32   Choroidal rupture due to contusion of the globe. A large arcuate and several vertical white ruptures run parallel to the disc margin. The choroid has disappeared in these areas and the bared sclera is visible. Blunt injury to the eye (12-year-old girl).

Fig 18-33   Macular hole after contusion of the globe. The margins of the defect are sharp and the defect looks punched out. The hole appears dark. It is oval due to traction by a scar (radial retinal folds). Vision: 5/35. Slingshot injury (14-year-old boy).

# 19. Ocular Changes in Black Patients

In general the same ocular diseases occur in black patients (with few exceptions) as seen in white patients living in the same area. With the exception of the background color of the fundus, the following illustrations show ocular changes similar to those seen in any other eye.

The following conditions will be illustrated: hypertensive retinopathy, lipemia retinalis, primary atrophy of the optic nerve, congenital toxoplasmosis and venous stasis retinopathy in cardiovascular hypertension. The picture of the anterior segment shows an ocular sarcoidosis which occurs more frequently among black than white patients.

Fig 19-1  Hypertensive retinopathy in a black patient (Thiel
III and IV). Mild disc edema. Pronounced attenuation of the retinal vessels. Numerous cotton-
wool deposits around the optic
nerve head extending into the
periphery. Blood pressure of
220/120 mmHg (58-year-old
man).

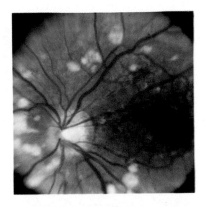

Fig 19-2  Lipemia retinalis in a
black patient. All retinal vessels
are filled by a milky yellow-red
fluid. This is a metabolic disorder
(hyperlipo-proteinemia) with
highly elevated triglycerol levels
in the serum (32-year-old man).

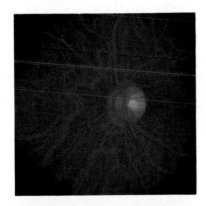

Fig 19-3  Primary atrophy of the
optic nerve in a black patient.
The optic nerve head is sharply
delineated and pale, especially
on the temporal side. The retinal
arterioles are attenuated and the
macular venules tortuous. Primary atrophy of the optic nerve after fracture of the skull
(18-year-old man).

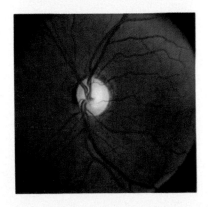

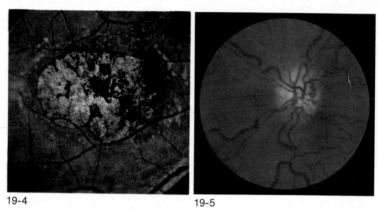

19-4                         19-5

Fig 19-4   Toxoplasmosis in the macula of a black patient ("rosette focus" of François in congenital toxoplasmosis). The large scar is yellow-green and involves the choroid and retina. It is surrounded by jet black hyperpigmentation. The retinal vessels course over the scar (26-year-old woman).

Fig 19-5   Venous stasis retinopathy in a black patient with cardiovascular hypertension and aortic stenosis. The retinal veins are dilated and tortuous. The arteries are attenuated and show a glistening reflex. The superior and inferior temporal vein show at 2 and at 7 o'clock a conspicuous S-shaped deviation because of the adjacent artery. There the two vessels are surrounded by a common adventitia. The disc and peripapillary area are edematous with newly formed blood vessels nasally. The macular venules are markedly tortuous. Blood pressure of 160/120 mmHg (48-year-old woman).

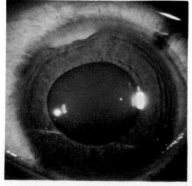

Fig 19-6   Iridocyclitis due to sarcoidosis in a black patient. The limbus is surrounded by a ring of pigmentation which is especially conspicuous between 2 and 7 o'clock. A white-yellow nodule lies in the chamber angle between 10:30 and 12 o'clock. The nodule pushes the root of the iris forward. The pupil is dilated (atropine). Histologic examination of a swollen regional lymph node revealed a noncaseating granulomatous inflammation. Sarcoidosis is found more frequently in black than in white patients (15-year-old boy).

# Index